بِسْمِ اللهِ الرَّحْمٰنِ الرَّحِيمِ

Clinical Manual of Hijama Therapy

By Dr. Feroz Osman-Latib

ISBN-13: 978-0-9911455-4-6

www.drlatib.com
email: info@drlatib.com

Ordering Information:
Quantity sales. Special discounts are available on quantity
purchases by bookstore, associations, and others. For
details, contact the publisher at the address above.

CONTENTS

Introduction	1
Cupping, Hijamah or Bloodletting	3
History of Hijamah	4
Ahadeeth on Hijamah	**8**
Virtues of Hijamah	8
Reasons for having Hijamah	9
Injury	9
Headaches	10
Sihr (black magic)	10
Poison	10
Paying the Hajjaam	10
The issue of Ijazah	11
Types of Hijamah / Bloodletting	**12**
Hijamah in the condition of strength	12
Days for performing Hijamah in strength	14
Hijamah in illness	15
Phlebotomy vs Hijamah	15
The effects of Hijamah on the body	**17**
Common effects of Hijamah	17
Effects of Hijamah as per Unani-Tibb	18
Hijamah's effects within the traditional Chinese medicine paradigm:	19
Modern Medical Understanding of Hijamah	21
Composition of the blood removed in Hijamah	22
Circulatory system effects	24
Effects on blood markers	25
Effect of Hijamah on the organs and systems	27
Effect of Hijamah on particular diseases	29
Taiba theory	**32**

Guidelines for performing Hijamah   34

Who should practice Hijamah ⋯⋯⋯⋯⋯⋯⋯⋯ 34
General contraindications and precautions ⋯⋯⋯⋯ 35
Who should have Hijamah done ⋯⋯⋯⋯⋯⋯ 40
8 patterns of illness ⋯⋯⋯⋯⋯⋯⋯⋯⋯⋯ 43
Circulation issues ⋯⋯⋯⋯⋯⋯⋯⋯⋯⋯⋯ 44
The condition of the person having Hijamah ⋯⋯⋯ 45
When should Hijamah be performed? ⋯⋯⋯⋯⋯ 46
Hijamah in strength ⋯⋯⋯⋯⋯⋯⋯⋯⋯⋯ 46
Hijamah and the lunar cycle: ⋯⋯⋯⋯⋯⋯⋯ 47
Hijamah in illness ⋯⋯⋯⋯⋯⋯⋯⋯⋯⋯⋯ 48
Body areas for Hijamah ⋯⋯⋯⋯⋯⋯⋯⋯⋯ 48
Areas/points that should not be bled ⋯⋯⋯⋯⋯ 49
How much blood should be removed? ⋯⋯⋯⋯⋯ 50
What to do after Hijamah? ⋯⋯⋯⋯⋯⋯⋯⋯ 51

Hijama and bloodletting techniques   53

Hijama Equipment ⋯⋯⋯⋯⋯⋯⋯⋯⋯⋯⋯ 57
Preparing the patient for Hijama ⋯⋯⋯⋯⋯⋯ 59
Bleeding techniques ⋯⋯⋯⋯⋯⋯⋯⋯⋯⋯ 60
Technique guide: ⋯⋯⋯⋯⋯⋯⋯⋯⋯⋯⋯ 61

Hijama Points Guide   67

SCALP ⋯⋯⋯⋯⋯⋯⋯⋯⋯⋯⋯⋯⋯⋯⋯ 67
FACE ⋯⋯⋯⋯⋯⋯⋯⋯⋯⋯⋯⋯⋯⋯⋯ 74
NECK AND UPPER BACK ⋯⋯⋯⋯⋯⋯⋯⋯ 81
LOWER BACK ⋯⋯⋯⋯⋯⋯⋯⋯⋯⋯⋯⋯ 92
UPPER LIMB ⋯⋯⋯⋯⋯⋯⋯⋯⋯⋯⋯⋯ 95
CHEST AND ABDOMEN ⋯⋯⋯⋯⋯⋯⋯⋯⋯ 102
LOWER LIMB ⋯⋯⋯⋯⋯⋯⋯⋯⋯⋯⋯⋯ 108

Point selection guide   128

Foreword

(to the 1st Edition)

This is one of the first books explaining cupping in such detail, it will benefit the patient and the practitioner to understand all the details of Hijamah.

Thus this book is a basic hand book on the practice of Hijamah for the layman and the medical practitioner.

Certain sections, only the one with good medical knowledge will benefit whilst the layman can draw information from other parts.

Many answers to commonly asked questions are well documented. Questions such as:-

1) Who should practice Hijamah?
2) The Shar'i status of Hijamah?
3) Who should have Hijamah done?
4) When should Hijamah be done?
5) What to do after Hijamah?
6) and How it is basically done?

One can safely conclude that this is a highly skilled procedure to be done by an expert.

Also it is recommended, not jurisprudically Sunnat.

May Allaah reward Dr Feroz Latib for explaining this matter adequately and May Allaah continue using him for Deen.

A.H. Elias (Mufti) (رحمة الله عليه)
May Allaah elevate his stages
1434 - 2013

Preface

"Indeed the best of remedies you have is hijama"
- Saheeh al-Bukhari (5371)

All Praise is due to Allaah who gave us the Deen of Islaam and perfected it for us until the day of Qiyaamah. All praise is due to Allaah whom we cannot praise in the manner that He should be praised, He is as He has described Himself and His magnificence is such that it cannot even begin to be described by creation. All praise is due to Allaah who sent our Noble Nabi Muhammad ﷺ as a mercy and guidance for all mankind.

Allaah Subhanahu wa Ta'aala has chosen mercy for His creation, and because of this, His commands and the life shown to us by His Ambiyaa (AS) encompass all that is beneficial for the spiritual, physical and social aspects of a human being, and society in general. Islaam itself places great emphasis on good health and physical fitness as this allows for the performance of Ibaadat and other acts that are meritorious in the eyes of Allaah. For this reason there are numerous Ahadeeth related to good health, the treatment of illness, the use of herbal substances etc. Entire books have been devoted to these topics, and amongst these writings perhaps the most famous are the Ahadeeth regarding honey, hijamah and habbatul barakah (black seed); as a result these three find common use amongst faithful Muslims the world over who adopt it for general health and the treatment of many, if not all medical conditions.

When one examines the Ahadeeth closely however, one realizes that there is a deeper layer that alludes to the treatment, whether it be hijamah, black seed, honey or any other treatment, being prescribed on the basis of "differentiation" which in turn requires sound medical knowledge. **From other Ahadeeth the Fuqahaa also deduce that one should visit a doctor who is an "expert" in their field.**

This brings to mind a wise saying that is quoted often in the books of our great scholars:

"Half a doctor is a danger to your life, and half a scholar is a danger to your faith"

The truth is that Hijamah is a medical procedure that should be performed by someone who has sound medical knowledge and is able to understand not only how to perform the procedure but when to do so, who to do it for, and when not to perform it.

Many will not understand this, as they believe that "cupping" or Hijamah must be beneficial at ALL times and in ALL conditions and that it can never be harmful, since it is "Sunnah".

This view is not correct and is not supported by the Ahadeeth either as there are ahadeeth which advise certain conditions wherein Hijama will be harmful and others where it is advised that the treatment should match the disease.

The correct view is this:

Hijamah when done at its appropriate time and for the right person who is in the condition suited to Hijamah will enable healing and cure for that person.

The scholars of Islaam also advise that administering medicine requires medical expertise and should not be done by the layperson. Therefore, with regard to any medical treatment recommended by Rasulullaah (Sallallaahu Álayhi Wasallam), due to health and medical intricacies as well as most country laws that define the scope of practice of medicine and medical procedures, one must exercise caution and consult with a physician who is a qualified expert in that field. Similarly, **with regard to Hijamah, although it is strongly recommended by Rasulullaah (Sallallaahu Álayhi Wasallam) in numerous Ahaadeeth**, it will be necessary to consult with a qualified practitioner before undergoing Hijama and then have it performed by one who has adequate medical training. This may be a medical practitioner or a practitioner of complementary and alternative medicine, who is duly qualified and registered with the relevant authority in that country to practice or a person who has studied Hijama through a reliable teacher or institution where they have also learned the anatomy and physiology of the human body and also the common medical illnesses and how to diagnose them and when patients need to be referred for further checkups based on their signs and symptoms. They should also be able to differentiate when Hijama will be suitable and when not.

By doing so, one will gain the benefits of Hijamah without the inherent harm that exists in practicing Hijamah without complete knowledge of its intricacies.

This is one of the fundamental reasons why I have written my first book on Hijama, for the patient and practitioner alike to understand all the details regarding hijamah, so that it can be a means of cure and not a means of sickness. This clinical manual for Hijama practitioners has been expanded to include detailed information on the points of the body which can be used for Hijama and how to select and use them appropriately. However, I would recommend anyone interested or currently practicing Hijama to go further into the study of Islamic Medicine in order to learn the finer intricacies as well as the use of other methods of treatment and medicinals appropriate to the illness. For this reason I have developed and continue to teach the course in Islamic Medicine which is a detailed and comprehensive course that is suitable for health practitioners and those without medical training as well. (The course is available for enrolment at courses.drlatib.com)

Regarding this it is important to narrate the hadeeth of 'Amr ibn Suh'aib (RA) who on his father's authority, said that his grandfather reported the Messenger of Allah (ﷺ) said to this meaning: "Anyone who practises medicine when he is not known as a practitioner will be held responsible."

عَنْ عَمْرِو بْنِ شُعَيْبٍ، عَنْ أَبِيهِ، عَنْ جَدِّهِ، أَنَّ رَسُولَ اللّهِ صلى الله عليه وسلم قَالَ :
مَنْ تَطَبَّبَ وَلاَ يُعْلَمُ مِنْهُ طِبٌّ فَهُوَ ضَامِنٌ .

The above hadeeth which is regarded as Hasan (and not weak or fabricated) sounds as a warning to us. Nabi ﷺ in this hadeeth is warning us sternly that in order to practice medicine we should be duly qualified and trained or else we will be held responsible meaning we may be taken to task on the day of Qiyamah either for the wrongs and errors committed in practicing or in general for practicing without knowledge.

I have been studying and teaching various aspects of complementary medicine for the past 23 years, including acupuncture, Chinese herbal medicine, chiropractic, laser therapy etc. I have a formal qualification from the Australian College of Natural Medicine where I specialized in Chinese Medicine and Acupuncture. I completed my internship at the Guangxi University Hospital in Nanning, China where I also received additional training in gynecology and pediatrics. I have taught at the South Australian College of Natural Medicine and also at the University of the Western Cape in South Africa. As well as at the TIbb Institute of Unary Medicine.

Together with teaching, delivering seminars and having served at the Allied Health Professions Council of South Africa I have been practicing and teaching hijamah/cupping for the last 15 years.

In this time I have heard of many irresponsible practices being performed in the name of Hijamah, these have often led to many side-effects including but not limited to miscarriages, severe blood loss, permanent scarring etc. that can be experienced when Hijamah is done incorrectly and inappropriately.

Many well-meaning individuals have also sprung up in numerous countries who aggressively advertise Hijamah and perform it whilst ignoring its most basic principles, some doing it solely for monetary incentive. They seek to profit both from people's desire to practice on the "Sunnah", and the hope that the sick hold for finding a cure for their ailments. As a result of being ignorant of the finer details of Hijamah, they end up doing more harm than good.

It is my hope that by writing this guide, patients and practitioners alike will have adequate knowledge to use hijamah properly and gain the true benefits in this form of treatment, which when done correctly is like no other in terms of its healing effects on the body. **Those contemplating having it done will have a better understanding of when, how and if it should be performed in their case**, and those performing it will do so with sound knowledge and eliminate the serious side-effects inherent in its incorrect practice. They will then serve as a means for bringing this "Sunnah" treatment to many who are desperately in need of it.

This clinical manual is a complete guide to the practice of Hijamah for interested medical professionals. It discusses all the aspects of Hijamah in detail, and goes to explain the procedure and the points that can be used and how select them.

For further updates, visit my website and subscribe to my mailing list.

Dr Feroz Osman-Latib
www.DrLatib.com
Twitter: @DrLatib

Introduction

Hijamah (حجامة) comes from the Arabic root word حجم which means "to diminish in volume", and refers to the reduction in blood volume or to the vacuum effect used to draw blood from the body. In the case of the Ahaadeeth (sayings of the Prophet Muhammad ﷺ) regarding hijamah it refers to the drawing of blood from the body for therapeutic purposes, either to maintain health in the case of one who is not sick or to cure a specific illness or ailment.

The vacuum or sucking effect can be achieved by many different methods including sucking with the mouth directly over a cut or wound (as in the case of poisonous bites), using a leech to draw blood, the use of instruments such as animal horns as was done in ancient times, or the more modern methods of using bamboo, glass or plastic "cups", either with fire to create a vacuum for suction or a pump mechanism to create the negative pressure (vacuum).

The practice of applying a partial vacuum by these means causes the tissues beneath the cup to be drawn up and swell, thereby increasing blood flow to the affected area. This enhanced blood flow draws impurities and toxins away from the nearby tissues and organs towards the surface for elimination via the break in the skin layer created through the incisions made prior to the application of the "cup" or similar device.

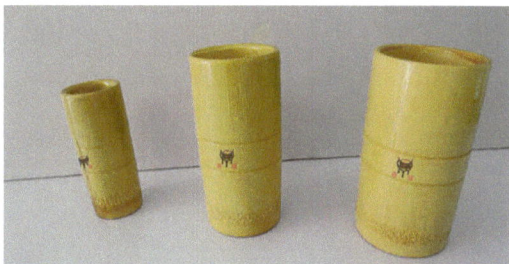

Bamboo cups were popular in Traditional Chinese Cupping before the arrival of plastic and glass cups. Many practitioners still prefer to use bamboo cups as they can be infused with an herbal decoction before application. Today it is not preferred for wet cupping as one cannot see the amount of blood being cupped and they are also impossible to sterilize properly since the bamboo may be porous.

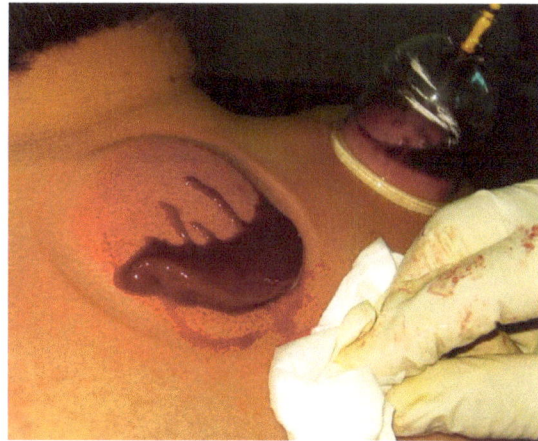

Nowadays disposable plastic cups are commonly used for the cupping procedure and represent a safe and affordable method of creating the vacuum needed. These cups however must be discarded after therapy, as the valve mechanism cannot be adequately sterilized. They should therefore only be used once. *(They should not be repeatedly used for the same patient either as is a common practice by some Hijama therapists)*

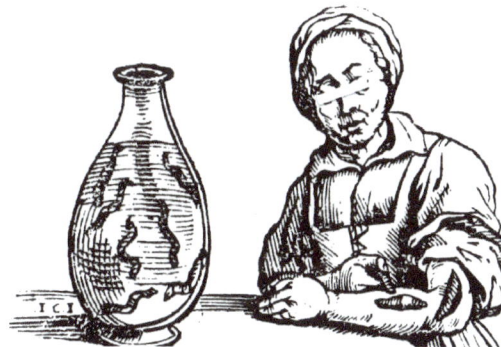

Leeches were also commonly used for drawing blood and have been approved by the FDA in the US for use in plastic and reconstructive surgery. These medicinal leeches are valued because while drawing blood they release natural anticoagulant and anesthetic substances and are therefore able to efficiently restore blood flow. Some cupping clinics employ the use of medicinal leeches and while it may be unpleasant it is in fact a safer and preferred option, which also leaves less scarring.

Though حجامة is commonly translated as "cupping" amongst English speakers, this is not an accurate translation because cupping in the modern sense can refer to both "dry" (where no blood is removed) and "wet" forms (which is حجامة). Cupping is the practice of using cups, which can be of different materials, to create suction at the skin level in order to draw blood to the surface, which may then be removed in the case of "wet" cupping.

Even amongst those who practice cupping, "wet" cupping is regarded the curative modality whereas dry cupping (in which no blood is removed), is more of a "relaxation therapy" and often practiced as part of relaxation massage techniques. Practitioners however do use dry cupping in order to "invigorate blood flow" in cases of blood "stasis"

While dry cupping has its uses, it is limited in its therapeutic effectiveness since the blood is drawn to the surface but not released, hence the effect of improving blood flow as well as release of some heat through the pores is achieved, but it is a temporary effect. Removing the blood in appropriate quantities from suitable locations and at the correct time will result in a much more effective and permanent treatment.

"Bloodletting" is the preferred term for حجامة and will be used throughout this book as it is more true to the meaning of Hijamah as implied by the Hadeeth. This is more so relevant since "cups" or similar instruments are not always used in the Hijamah procedure, as even an incision in the right part of the body intended to release blood from that area can be considered Hijamah, so can the use of leeches to draw blood. Both do not involve the use of cups, but are true to the essence of Hijamah. In fact there are Ahadeeth where the "blade of the Hajjaam" is mentioned as having the cure and is a indication that the act of releasing blood is the curative factor in Hijamah and not particularly the "mihjam" or instrument that is used to draw the blood.

In keeping with this understanding, the one who performs Hijamah will be referred to as the حجّام (Hajjaam) in this book.

It is recorded in the books of Ahadeeth that amongst other things, such as the use of the turban and miswak, hijamah was a practice of every Prophet (AS).

Considering that the Quran clearly states that every nation was sent a guide, and the narrations that approximately 124 000 or 200 000 Prophets (AS) were sent to this world, Hijamah as a treatment is to be found throughout the world as a result of this long history of continuous use. Indeed historical texts prove that this is the case with depictions of cupping equipment being seen on ancient stone tablets and markings from archeological findings throughout the world.

The earliest historical evidence of the use of Hijamah is from the ancient Egyptians. One of the oldest Egyptian medical textbooks, written in approximately 1550 BC (+-3500 years ago), describes "bleeding" used to 'remove pathogens from the body'. It is evident that bloodletting was considered a remedy for almost every type of disease as well as an important means of preserving good health and life.

Hippocrates and Galen were also great advocates of Hijamah. In Hippocrates' time bloodletting was topological and not used in terms of the theory of the 4 humors. Specific points were bled for specific illnesses. Galen explains that the principle indication for bloodletting is to eliminate residues or divert blood from one part of the body to another. His approach was based on two key Unani concepts prevalent at the time. **First, that blood did not circulate well in the body, and that it eventually went stagnant until it was "let out". Secondly, the concept of the balance of the four humors (blood, phlegm, black bile and yellow bile) was the source of health or illness, in which case bloodletting is used to bring about balance between these humors**. Mapping out the blood vessels of the body, Galen would cut his patients in different areas; depending on what area he wanted to treat.

In the middle east region we find that the practice of Hijamah was already present before the arrival of the final Rasul ﷺ and the final Nabi ﷺ both encouraged and used it himself on many occasions. **Ibn Sina, the famous physician said: 'Hijamah is not preferred in the beginning or the end of the month. It is preferred in the middle of the month when the substances (of the constitution or the condition) accumulate and become agitated**.

The Talmud included rules for days where bloodletting could be practiced and early Christian writings also outlined which days were the best for bloodletting therapy.

In the East, Bloodletting and wet cupping was always an integral part of the medical practices, and remains so to this day. The ancient Chinese medical text which is widely regarded as the oldest medical text in existence, the Nei Jing, or Inner Classic says that:
"if there is stagnation it must be first be

resolved through bloodletting before the application of acupuncture or moxibustion."

Another ancient Chinese medical text the Su Wen gives detailed instructions for piercing combined with bloodletting but forbidding the letting of blood in certain seasons.

The Su Wen states:

"When heaven is warm and when the sun is bright,
then the blood in man is rich in liquid and the protective qi (energy/lifeforce) is at the surface
Hence the blood can be drained easily, and the qi can be made to move on easily..."

Some researchers believe that acupuncture actually began as bloodletting, with sharp objects being used to bleed the acupuncture points before the widespread use of needles to perform acupuncture.
This is also evidenced by depictions of ancient "needles" which were more akin to bleeding instruments than the fine acupuncture needles in use today.

The Lingshu (Spiritual Pivot) and its companion volume, the Suwen (Simple Questions), written around 100 B.C., established the fundamentals of traditional Chinese medical ideas and acupuncture therapy. Originally, there was a set of 9 acupuncture needles, which included the triangular lance, sword-like flat needles, and fairly large needles. Regarding the fourth needle, which has a tubular body and lance-like tip, the text states: "This can be used to drain fevers, to draw blood, and to exhaust chronic diseases." The seventh needle is described as being hair fine (corresponding to modern acupuncture needles); it is said to "control fever and chills and painful rheumatism in the luo channels." In modern practice, using the lance as a means to treat chronic diseases has been marginalized (except to treat acute flare-ups of chronic ailments), while the applications of the hair-fine needle has been greatly expanded beyond malarial fevers and muscle and joint pain.

Traditional Chinese Medicine and Acupuncture practitioners still use bleeding therapies though it is more commonly practiced in China than by western practitioners due to concerns about infection and the general dislike for dealing with blood in the acupuncture clinic.

North American natives are reported to have used buffalo horns for wet cupping. The horns were hollowed with a small hole at the top through which the cupper would suck the air out of, in order to create a vacuum in the horn which would then pull up the blood from the incisions previously made with a blade.

Buffalo horns are also reported as being used for Hijamah during the Babylon - Assyrian Empire (stretching from Iraq to the Mediterranean).

Bloodletting became widespread during the middle ages and surprisingly, became a practice common to barbers who would display a "bloodletting pole" outside their establishment to indicate that they practiced bloodletting.

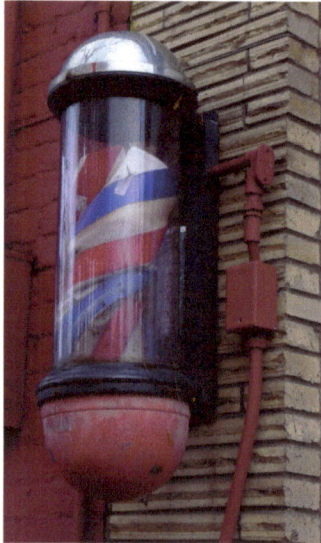

In this way it also became widespread in the US due to colonial influence from Europe and as a matter of fact, George Washington, the first U.S. president, died as a result of erroneously performed bloodletting. He had close to 4 liters of blood removed from his body on the same day as a supposed treatment for an infection and died as a result of excessive blood loss.

The traditional principles of Hijamah were largely being ignored during this time with the procedure being carried out incorrectly by barbers who had no medical knowledge and therefore resulted in a large number of adverse effects and even many unnecessary deaths.

In Europe, the main process of bloodletting in the 19th century as performed by those in the medical establishment included the use of leeches to drain blood from a patient. France reportedly imported approximately 40 million leeches for the purpose of bloodletting during this period.

In Finland, medicinal bleeding has been practiced at least since the 15th century, and it is still done traditionally in saunas. Cups made of cow's horns were commonly used. These had a valve mechanism in it to create the negative pressure within the cup for suction to take place. (Wet cupping is still commonly used in Finland as a complementary/alternative medicine.)

By the mid to late 1800's however, bloodletting was sharply criticized by the medical fraternity and had fallen away as a popular method. Because of the procedure not being practiced correctly it was becoming responsible for a large number of deaths and therefore was increasingly being discredited by modern medicine, the newly established scientific model of medicine also began discrediting all other previously established traditional therapies in order to gain medical dominance.

There were valid concerns regarding the practice as well and in 1828, Pierre Charles Alexandre Louis openly criticized bloodletting for the treatment of diseases. His research found that in patients with pneumonia, 44% of those who were bled within the first four days died, compared with 25% of those patients who were bled later in their illness. He deduced that bloodletting was not useful in the treatment of pneumonia.

Bloodletting managed to survive however into the first part of the 20th century; it was even recommended in a 1923 edition of a textbook called The Principles and Practice of Medicine. During those days, there were four main bloodletting methods practiced by physicians. The first was the continued use of leeches as a bloodletting modality. The second was bleeding of superficial arteries. The third was phlebotomy (also known as "breathing a vein") where a large external vein would be cut in order to draw blood and the last was scarification – a method which involved using tools to make multiple incisions in the skin from which blood was drawn through "cupping".

As the 20th century brought new medical knowledge, technology and scientific research based validation (and negation) of medical practices, bloodletting died out in modern medicine in the western world almost entirely within a few decades. It remained very much still a part of Chinese (and Japanese) Medical therapy, though practitioners trained outside of China or Japan were reluctant to perform the procedure. It also remained in use in the Muslim world including the Middle East and countries with larger Muslim populations such as Indonesia, Malaysia etc.

In the past 20 to 30 years it has found a tremendous resurgence amongst Muslim communities living in other parts of the world as well, with courses being offered to both medical practitioners and the public in many countries.

In most western countries however like the US, Canada and Australia, medical law does not permit the practice of Hijamah by a non-medical trained individual though the practice may still exist informally amongst certain ethnic and religious communities.

Since it involves piercing of the skin and exposure to blood and other body fluids and there is therefore a high risk of spreading of infections such as HIV and Hepatitis, not to mention the possibility of serious side effects, authorities in these countries have appropriately seen fit to legislate its use to qualified and registered health practitioners such as acupuncturists, medical practitioners etc.

The books of Ahaadeeth, which are the sayings and also the practices of the Nabi Muhammad (ﷺ) as recorded by his illustrious companions (RA) are replete with the mention of Hijamah describing its virtues and giving advice about when it is to be performed etc. In this section I will mention only the Ahadeeth regarding its virtues and also the hadith indicating the permissibility of paying a fee for the treatment. The Ahadeeth regarding payment are mentioned because there are many of the belief that there should be no payment for Hijamah whereas this is against the Sunnah of the Nabi ﷺ. Other Ahadeeth regarding the specific matters of Hijamah will be discussed in their relevant chapters.

Virtues of Hijamah

*Jabir bin Abdullaah (RA) relates that he heard Rasulullaah ﷺ saying: "If there is any good in your treatments **it is in the blade of the Hajjaam**, a drink of honey or branding by fire (cauterization), **whichever suits the ailment**, and I do not like to be cauterized" (Bukhari and Muslim)*

Asim b. 'Umar b. Qatada reported: There came to our house 'Abdullaah and another person from amongst the members of the household who complained of a wound. Jabir said: What ails you? He said: There is a wound which is very painful for me, whereupon he said: Lad, bring to me a hajjaam. He said: 'Abdullaah, what do you intend to do with the Hajjaam? I said: I would get this wound

*cupped. He said: By Allaah, even the touch of a fly or cloth causes me pain (and cupping) would thus cause me (unbearable) pain. And when he saw him feeling pain (at the idea of Hijamah), he said: I heard Allaah's Rasul (may peace be upon him) as saying: **If there is any effective remedy amongst your remedies, these are (three): Hijamah, drinking of honey and cauterization with the help of fire**. Allaah's Rasul (may peace be upon him) had said: As for myself I do not like cauterization. The Hajjaam was called and he cupped him and he was alright. (Sahih Muslim 26:5468)*

*Narrated By Abu Hurayrah (RA): Abu Hind cupped the Nabi ﷺ in the middle of his head. The Nabi ﷺ said: Banu Bayadah, marry Abu Hind (to your daughter), and ask him to marry (his daughter) to you. He said: **The best thing by which you treat yourself is Hijamah**. (Abu Dawud 5:2097)*

*Narrated By Abu Hurayrah: The Nabi (pbuh) said: **The best medical treatment you apply is Hijamah**. (Abu Dawud 22:3848)*

*Abu Hurairah (RA) narrates that Rasulullaah ﷺ said: "**Whoever has hijamah done on the 17th, 19th or 21st of the month, it will be for him a cure from every illness**" (Sahih Al-Jaami' 5968)*

*Abu Hurairah (RA) narrates that Rasulullaah ﷺ said: "Jibra'eel conveyed to me that **the best amongst the things that mankind uses for treatment is hijamah**" (Sahih Al-Jaami 213)*

Abdullaah ibn Abbas (RA) reported that the

Rasul ﷺ said, "I did not pass by an angel from the angels on the night journey except that they all said to me: **Upon you is Hijamah, O Muhammad.**" [Saheeh Sunan ibn Maajah (3477).

In the narration reported by Abdullaah ibn Mas'ud (RA) the angels said, **"Oh Muhammad, order your Ummah (nation) with Hijamah."** [Saheeh Sunan Tirmidhi (3479)]

Rasulullaah (Sallallaahu Álayhi Wasallam) said, 'Jibraaeel (Álayhis salaam) **repeatedly emphasized upon me to resort to Hijamah** to the extent that I feared that Hijamah will be made compulsory.' (Jamúl Wasaail p. 179).

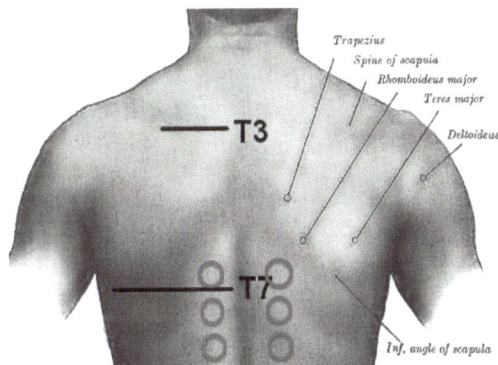

Rasulullaah (Sallallaahu Álayhi Wasallam) praised a person who performs Hijamah, saying **it removes blood, lightens the back and sharpens the eyesight** (Jamúl Wasaail p. 179)

Hadhrat Abu Kabsha (Radhiallaahu Ánhu) narrates that Rasulullaah (Sallallaahu Álayhi Wasallam) used to undergo cupping on the head and between his shoulders and he used to say, '**Whosoever removes this blood, it will not harm him that he**

does not take any other medical treatment.' (Mishkãt p. 389)

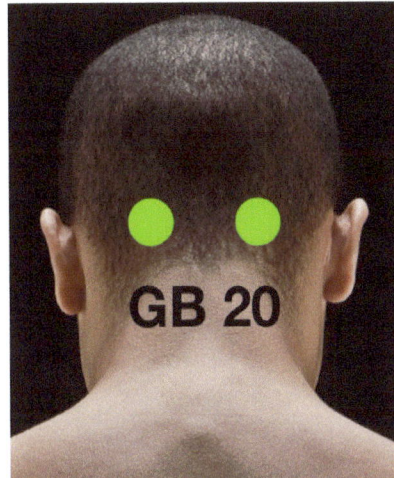

Reasons for having Hijamah

Besides the general effects of Hijamah in improving and maintaining good health, especially in the hot regions, the Nabi ﷺ also used and recommended Hijamah for specific illnesses.

Injury

Jaabir ibn Abdullaah (RA) reported that the Rasul ﷺ fell from his horse onto the trunk of a palm tree and dislocated his foot. Waki' (RA) said, "Meaning the Rasul ﷺ **was cupped on (his foot) for bruising.**" [Saheeh Sunan ibn Maajah (2807)].

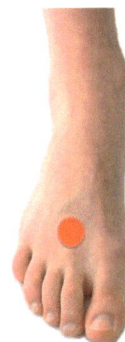

Headaches

سَلْمَى خَادِمِ رَسُولِ اللَّهِ صلى الله عليه وسلم قَالَتْ
مَا كَانَ أَحَدٌ يَشْتَكِي إِلَى رَسُولِ اللَّهِ صلى الله عليه
وسلم وَجَعًا فِي رَأْسِهِ إِلاَّ قَالَ " احْتَجِمْ " . وَلاَ وَجَعًا
فِي رِجْلَيْهِ إِلاَّ قَالَ " اخْضِبْهُمَا "

Salma (RA), the servant of the Rasul ﷺ said, "**Whenever someone would complain of a headache to the Rasul of Allaah ﷺ, he ﷺ would advise them to perform Hijamah.**" [Saheeh Sunan abi Dawud (3858)].

Sihr (black magic)

Ibn al-Qaiyum (RA) mentions that the Rasul ﷺ **was cupped on his head when he was afflicted with sihr** and that it is from the best of cures for this if performed correctly. [Zaad al Ma'aad (4/125-126)].

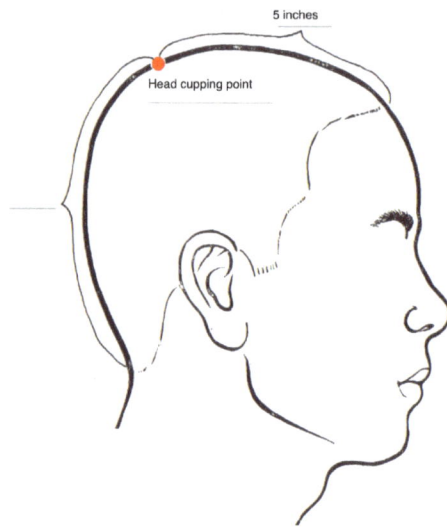

Poison

Abdullaah ibn Abbas (RA) reported that a Jewish woman gave poisoned meat to the Rasul ﷺ so he ﷺ sent her a message saying, "What caused you to do that?" She replied, "If you really are a Nabi then Allaah will inform you of it and if you are not then I would save the people from you!" **When the Rasul ﷺ felt pain from it, he ﷺ performed Hijamah. Once he travelled while in Ihram and felt that pain and hence performed hijamah.** [Ahmed (1/305) the Hadeeth is Hasan].

These four conditions mentioned in the Ahadeeth for which the Nabi ﷺ had Hijamah done give us an indication as to what type of diseases Hijamah is useful for viz.:

1. External injuries
2. Internal disorders which are either due to heat, poor circulation or build up of toxins
3. Sihr (black magic)
4. Poison (this can also be commonly ingested "poisons" which are taken indeliberatley without being aware of them being poisons such as heavy metal ingestion from mercury fillings and also minute plastics which have now been found to be present in human beings)

Paying the Hajjaam

فَقَالَ أَنَسٌ احْتَجَمَ رَسُولُ اللَّهِ صلى الله عليه وسلم
وَحَجَمَهُ أَبُو طَيْبَةَ فَأَمَرَ لَهُ بِصَاعَيْنِ مِنْ طَعَامٍ وَكَلَّمَ
أَهْلَهُ فَوَضَعُوا عَنْهُ مِنْ خَرَاجِهِ وَقَالَ " إِنَّ أَفْضَلَ مَا
تَدَاوَيْتُمْ بِهِ الْحِجَامَةُ " . أَوْ " إِنَّ مِنْ أَمْثَلِ دَوَائِكُمُ
الْحِجَامَةَ " . قَالَ وَفِي الْبَابِ عَنْ عَلِيٍّ وَابْنِ عَبَّاسٍ
وَابْنِ عُمَرَ . قَالَ أَبُو عِيسَى حَدِيثُ أَنَسٍ حَدِيثٌ حَسَنٌ
صَحِيحٌ . وَقَدْ رَخَّصَ بَعْضُ أَهْلِ الْعِلْمِ مِنْ أَصْحَابِ
النَّبِيِّ صلى الله عليه وسلم وَغَيْرِهِمْ فِي كَسْبِ
الْحَجَّامِ . وَهُوَ قَوْلُ الشَّافِعِيِّ .

Narrated Anas:

"The Messenger of Allah (ﷺ) was cupped. Abu Talhah did the cupping. So he ordered that he be given two Sa' of food, and he spoke to his masters to reduce his taxes. He said: 'The most virtuous of what you treat with is cupping.' Or, he said: 'The best of your treatments is cupping.'" [He said:] There are narrations on this topic from 'Ali, Ibn 'Abbas, and Ibn 'Umar. [Abu 'Eisa said:] The Hadith of Anas is a Hasan Sahih. Some of the people of knowledge among the Companions of the Prophet (ﷺ), and others permitted paying the cupper. This is the view of Ash-Shafi'i.

Anas RadiyAllaahu'Anhu was asked regarding the payment to a hajjaam. (Is it permissible or not?) Anas RadiyAllaahu 'Anhu replied: "Rasulullaah SallAllaahu 'Alayhi Wasallam took the treatment of Hijamah which was administered by Abu Taybah RadiyAllaahu 'Anhu, **he was given two saa' food** *(in a narration it is mentioned that dates were given), and Sayyidina Rasulullaah SallAllaahu'Alayhi Wasallam interceded on his behalf to his master that the stipulated amount he was responsible for be made less. He also said this, that Hijamah is the best of medicine".(Tirmidhi 49:001)*

'Ali RadiyAllaahu 'Anhu reports: "Rasulullaah SallAllaahu 'Alayhi Wasallam once took the treatment of Hijamah **and asked me to pay its fees. I paid the hajjaam his fees"**. *(Tirmidhi 49:002)*

Ibn 'Abbaas RadiyAllaahu 'Anhu said that Rasulullaah SallAllaahu 'Alayhi Wasallam took the treatment of Hijamah on both sides

of his neck and between his shoulders, **and paid the hajjaam his fees. If it had been haraam, he would not have paid it**. *(Tirmidhi 49:003)*

The issue of Ijazah

Some books vehemently oppose the performing of Hijamah without "Ijazah", which literally means "permission" and refers to the granting of such permission by a teacher or sheikh to a student that he deems fit to perform the practice. This is a nonsensical idea and a clear error. If this were true then who gave "Ijazah" to the slave who performed Hijamah for the Nabi ﷺ? The fact is that Hijamah was already being practiced before Islaam, and in fact there is a reference to this in the hadith where the Nabi ﷺ says "the best of **your** medicine is Hijamah". Some scholars mention that "your" in the hadith is an indication that this was already a practice of the people of Hijaz.

The truth is that **"Ijazah" is not needed to perform Hijamah, but rather sound knowledge of its method and principles are needed**. The benefits of Hijamah will be attained irrespective of whether the person performing it is a sheikh or even a Muslim. Yes, it is better that a pious Muslim practitioner performs the procedure but it is not an essential aspect of Hijamah or gaining its benefits.

There are a number of different methods and types of bloodletting. The Hajjaam should know in detail which method is best, based on:

• the patients health and general constitution
• the presenting ailment
• geographic, seasonal and climatic factors

It is essential that a Hajjaam is trained in the above aspects in order to know when to do Hijama and more importantly when not to do Hijama.

(These matters are discussed in further detail in my courses available at my website)

Hijamah in the condition of strength

The simplest method of Hijamah is that used for general health promotion. In this type of Hijamah there is no serious complaint by the patient that would warrant a special type of Hijamah or the use of "special" Hijamah points other than the standard points on the back, neck or head. This is traditionally termed as Hijamah-bi-Sihhat (Hijamah in the condition of health), many also refer to it as "sunnah cupping". Both terms are not correct however as the Rasul of Allaah ﷺ had cupping done both in health and as a treatment for particular pains and ailments, and it is also rare to find someone nowadays with absolutely no illness. I prefer the term Hijamah in strength, referring to performing Hijamah for someone who is of general good health

and strength.
Such a patient may however complain of general symptoms such as a feeling of sluggishness, tiredness etc, they may also have a regular habit of doing Hijamah and are aware of the benefits it has for them personally, or they are trying this method of health preservation for the first time under recommendation from their friends or acquaintances.

Basically their general health is good, and very importantly their pulse is strong indicating a healthy amount of blood and also a good amount of heat in the blood. (They could also be suffering from a constitutional blood or heat excess as is common in hot climates.)

If the pulse is weak or deep then this type of Hijamah may be contraindicated as this means that there is less blood or that the heat of the body is internal and not in the exterior parts of the body.

In this type of Hijamah care is taken to observe the rules of Hijamah with regard to the condition of the patient, as well as the season, climate, day of the lunar month and time of the day in which Hijamah is performed as this greatly influences the nature of blood that will be removed. **Not observing these and performing this type of general Hijamah outside of its recommended times will not result in any benefit for the patient and will very often result in long term harm for the patients health**. This may not be apparent immediately after the procedure, but will be noticed in the months and even years to come afterward.

When applying Hijamah in the condition of strength the areas being cupped are standard, these are mentioned in the Ahadeeth:

Hadhrat Abu Kabsha (Radhiallaahu Ánhu) narrates that Rasulullaah (Sallallaahu Álayhi Wasallam) used to undergo cupping on the **head and between his shoulders** and he used to say, 'Whosoever removes this blood, it will not harm him that he does not take any other medical treatment.' (Mishkãt p. 389)

It is apparent that what is meant in this hadeeth is in regards to health maintenance, not the treatment of a specific illness.

From examining the various Ahadeeth and by consensus of those experienced practitioners of Hijamah the areas used in this general form of Hijamah are detailed in the sections to follow but briefly they are:

For a man:

1. The area between the shoulder blades, most commonly in line with the inferior end of the scapula which is in line with the 7th thoracic vertebra. Sometimes other points lateral to the spinal column between the spinouts processes of the 6th to 9th thoracic vertebrae are used. This particular area is the best for performing general Hijamah as it is the area where toxins and impurities in the blood accumulate and stagnate especially around the 17th. 19th and 21st of the month.

2. The occipital area of the neck in the recesses formed between the upper portion of the sternocleidomastoid and the trapezius muscles. Treating this area is helpful in resolving a number of common ailments of the head and neck, including headache, vertigo, pain/stiffness of neck, blurry vision, red/painful eyes, tinnitus, nasal obstruction, common cold, and rhinorrhea (runny nose, nasal discharge associated with allergies or hay fever or common cold). It's also very useful for insomnia, and tends to have a relaxing and balancing effect upon the nervous system.

3. On the head in the midline and at the intersection of aline drawn from he apex of each ear.

4. On the anterior aspect of the foot in a depression distal to the junction of the 2nd and 3rd metatarsal bones. This area is traditionally used to treat swelling, headache, dizziness / vertigo, abdominal pain, bloating, constipation. It can also aid groundedness and focus and treat ADD/ADHD, mania, restlessness, palpitations and epilepsy.

In women the same areas are used except for the Hijamah point on the head but the quantity of blood removed is less. Note that women are not in need of regular Hijamah as they do release blood through the menses, if they have experienced menopause then it is fine to do as long as they are still strong and not suffering from blood deficiency in which case one must observe the rules of performing Hijamah in illness.

Days for performing Hijamah in strength

Anas ibn Maalik (RA) reported that the Rasul ﷺ said, "**Whoever wants to perform Hijamah then let him search for the 17th, 19th and 21st...**" [Saheeh Sunan ibn Maajah (3486)].

These are the generally accepted dates for Hijamah in strength, irrespective of what day of the week they fall on, though there are other Ahadeeth that seem to prohibit having it done on particular days of the week, though Imam Malik says that it cannot be performed on any day.

Ibn Umar (RA) reported that the Rasul ﷺ said, "Hijamah on an empty stomach is best. In it is a cure and a blessing. It improves the intellect and the memory. So cup yourselves with the blessing of Allaah on Thursday. Keep away from Hijamah on Wednesday, Friday, Saturday and Sunday to be safe. Perform Hijama on Monday and Tuesday for it is the day that Allaah saved Ayoub from a trial. He was inflicted with the trial on Wednesday. You will not find leprosy except (by being cupped) on Wednesday or Wednesday night." [Sunan ibn Maajah (3487)].

Ibn Umar (RA) reported that the Rasul ﷺ said, "Hijamah on an empty stomach is best. It increases the intellect and improves the memory. It improves the memory of the one memorising. So whoever is going to be cupped then (let it be) on a Thursday in the name of Allaah. Keep away from being cupped on a Friday, Saturday and Sunday. Be cupped on a Monday or Tuesday. Do not be cupped on a Wednesday because it is the day that Ayoub was befallen with a trial. You will not find leprosy except (by being cupped) on Wednesday or Wednesday night." [Sunan ibn Maajah (3488)].

In reconciling these it can be said that for Hijamah in strength, the dates are specified, they are the 17th, 19th or 21st of the lunar month and the best is when these dates coincide with a Monday, Tuesday or Thursday, though there is no prohibition for having this type of Hijamah done on any other day as long as it corresponds with the 17th, 19th and 21st.

(There is difference of opinion regarding the prohibition on particular days of the week, since another way of reconciling is considering that the Nabi of Allaah ﷺ in the above two Ahadeeth was referring to that particular month in which the Hadeeth was narrated and referring directly to the days of that week and the week after. If Thursday was the 19th, then the previous Friday, Saturday and Sunday would be the 13th, 14th and 15th, and on these days of the Islaamic month it is mentioned that cupping should not be done, Monday and Tuesday would be the 16th and 17th which would be okay for cupping, since they are after the full moon. Wednesday being prohibited in this case would be the exact day of the year that corresponded with the illness of Nabi Ayyoob (AS), and Thursday being the ideal day to perform Hijamah.)

It is important to note that this type of Hijamah (i,.e Hijamah in strength / Sunnah Hijamah) should preferably be performed only in the seasons of spring and summer. When the climate is hot. However, in places like Hejaz where it is hot throughout the year it can also be performed in the other seasons.

Further detail is discussed in the chapters on the guidelines for performing Hijamah.

Hijamah in illness

When a patient is complaining of a particular condition, i.e. they are not in good health, but suffering from a particular illness for which Hijamah is indicated then this is termed Hijama-bil-Mardh (Hijamah in illness).

In illness the rules of Hijamah are different. For this reason Imam Ahmad ibn Hanbal would have Hijamah at any time of the month and hour of the day as a result of the need of performing Hijamah due to illness. When performing Hijamah for a specific illness it should be done at those points of the body indicated for the illness and the rules of the amount of blood being removed etc. should be adhered to for maximum benefit. These are discussed in the Hijamah treatment guide. This type of Hijamah is very specialized and involves three major aspects:-

1. Diagnosing the individual and the sickness correctly
2. The correct selection of points (or superficial veins) to bleed,
3. Removing the correct amount of blood in

order to effect cure of the patient's illness.

It is also highly recommended to use herbal preparations in association with the Hijamah to address deficiencies/excesses present and treat cold or heat that is present. (for more information on Islamic herbal remedies that can be used in conjunction please see my website www.drlatib.com)

Phlebotomy vs Hijamah

Phlebotomy is often confused with Hijamah yet the two are very different in their method and effect on the body. Phlebotomy is the bleeding of veins via the use of a hypodermic needle and results in releasing of blood from the inner parts of the body as opposed to the outer part which is achieved through traditional Hijamah. It will also be regarded as part of bloodletting, but not Hijamah in the sense as described by the Prophet ﷺ, as there are significant differences in the use of these two types of bloodletting.

To understand the difference it is important to remember that the land of Hijaaz (wherefrom the Ahadeeth of Hijamah are reported) is generally a hot and dry region.

Hot versus cold climates have different effects on the blood flow and distribution in the body. In hot countries, and other countries in the hot season, the blood and therefore heat of the body flows strongly within the outer part of the body, whilst the inner parts remain cooler and relatively deficient of blood.

For this reason perspiration increases in summer, i.e in order to regulate body temperature, and because of the inner organs being cooler, foods take longer to digest, and many summer-heat type illnesses occur.

In cold countries, and in winter, the blood and resultant heat of a person's body goes to the inner portions. As a result the digestive system is strengthened, more sleep is experienced, and food is digested easily.

For this reason rich foods digest easily in winter, and take more time in summer. This is also the reason honey; dates and other heat creating foods do not affect the people of Hijaaz as they do in other countries with colder climates.

In Hijamah, the blood in the outer parts of the body is removed, this is the peripheral circulation and in Hijaaz the heat is more

on the outer parts of the body, therefore, Hijamah is more beneficial in hot countries and hot climates.

In phlebotomy blood is let from the veins and therefore reduces heat from the inner parts of the body, therefore it will not be beneficial in hot countries and climates and was hence not a practice of the Nabi ﷺ and the people of Hijaz.

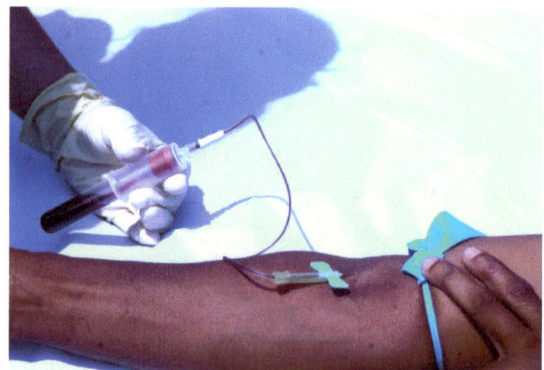

Drawing blood from the veins beneath the superficial skin layer is considered phlebotomy and does not have the same effect as traditional Hijamah

The simplest explanation of Hijamah's effects is the removal of "bad" blood or impurities from the blood.

This is a common explanation whether it is from the Indians of North America to lay practitioners in western countries.

Some may also use it for its ability to remove the effects of "sihr" or "black magic" as well as "nazr" or the "evil eye".

Common effects of Hijamah

1. Removal of "bad" blood or impurities from the blood
2. Treatment of Sihr (black magic) or Nazr (evil eye)

There are other effects that are explained in more detail in a number of traditional medical systems as well as through modern scientific research. Understanding these is important as it allows for the correct selection and application of Hijamah techniques depending on the patient and the illness they are presenting with.

Amongst the traditional medical paradigms, Unani-Tibb and Traditional Chinese Medicine are the most detailed in terms of understanding why and how Hijamah works in maintaining health and treating illness. Unani-Tibb is practiced in the Graeco-Arab region as well as by Unani practitioners throughout the world. Traditional Chinese Medicine is practiced in the Asian regions and also by practitioners throughout the world and these two have similar philosophies with regards to the effect of Hijamah.

Unani-tibb is a form of traditional medicine widely practiced by Muslims and is largely based on the teachings of the Greek physician Hippocrates, and Roman physician Galen, which was developed into an elaborate medical System by Arab and Persian physicians, such as al-Razi, Ibn Sena, Al-Zahrawi, and Ibn Nafis. **Muslim practitioners are referred to as a Hakim**.

Unani philosophy is based on the concept of the four humors: Phlegm (Balgham), Blood (Dam), Yellow bile (Safrā') and Black bile (Saudā'). It maintains that disease occurs through imbalance, or contamination, of these 4 humors, or alternatively as a result of the body being weak. It is very much concerned with the temperament of the body and considers aspects such as heat, coolness, dryness, phlegm and moisture and how these cause and contribute to illness. Bloodletting acts to remove contamination in the blood, rebalance the humors and draws excessive heat out of the body. In the case of traditional Hijamah (as opposed to phlebotomy) this heat will be drawn from the outer parts of the body, though there are indirect effects on the internal organs and systems.

Contemporary Unani practitioners believe that Hijamah acts to draw inflammation and pressure away from the deep organs (especially the heart, brain, lungs, liver and kidneys) towards the skin. This facilitates the healing process. They also explain that this process strengthens the immune system, encouraging the optimum functioning of the body by assisting the actions of "Physis". It diverts toxins and other harmful impurities from these vital organs towards the "less-vital" skin, before expulsion. The blood that is diverted also then allows for a fresh 'stream' of blood to that area.

Effects of Hijamah as per Unani-Tibb

3. Diverts and expels toxins and harmful impurities from the vital organs
4. Removes excess blood
5. Removes excess heat from the blood and surface of the body
6. Draws inflammation away from the deeper organs
7. Assists the body's own healing abilities

Traditional Chinese Medicine(TCM) is similar to Unani-Tibb in its concept of "Humors", though in the case of TCM it is the balance of 5 phases/elements viz. water, fire, wood, earth and metal and their correspondences in the body. TCM however also adds the concept of proper movement and flow of blood and "qi" throughout the body. Qi is the vital energy of the body that is responsible for directing all the body's functions. It moves within the blood and it also moves the blood itself. Qi is present in different forms, it includes but is not limited to the energy of the heart and lungs as they contract and expand, the force of the muscles in the body that open

and close the various sphincters and also allow for bodily movement. It is also responsible for many phenomena of the body that would be attributed to the "soul" and even the "nafs" and is something that permeates the entire body but departs when a person dies, whereas the blood and form of the body remains.

In Traditional Chinese Medicine, it is believed that health is maintained when the blood and "qi" flow smoothly throughout the body. When there is stagnation or stasis this leads to disease which can be systemic, affecting the whole body, or local, affecting a particular organ or part of the body. Hijamah is particularly effective at relieving this "stasis" and acts to restore proper flow especially of blood but also of qi in the body or local region

Stagnation or stasis is not the only pathology however that Hijamah treats within TCM. In TCM there is a disease differentiation system called the 8 patterns. In this system it is determined whether a disease is internal or external, hot or cold, excess or deficient and yin or yang. This matrix is then used to determine the core nature of an illness.

When this system produces a pattern that is excess and heat related then Hijamah is indicated. Excess heat patterns include Internal pathologies such as blood heat, blood toxins, liver heat, heat rising up in the body, stomach fire, large intestine fire, heart fire etc. and can be effectively addressed by حجامة or bloodletting. These patterns are characteristically defined by their being an "internal", "excess", "hot" pattern of disease.

"External" excess heat patterns correspond with febrile infectious diseases and can also be effectively addressed by bloodletting. These include traditional Chinese medicine patterns such as invasion of wind-heat, toxic heat, spring warm etc.

Normally Hijamah is not indicated when there is a deficient heat pattern of any type, or a cold pattern except where there is significant stagnation. If it is used in these cases only a small amount of blood is removed so as not to worsen the "deficiency" or "cold" aspect of the disease.

In terms of the deeper principles of yin and yang, bleeding can also be used in cases of blood deficiency. For these cases a small amount of blood is removed which then has the effect of stimulating blood production.

Hijamah's effects within the traditional Chinese medicine paradigm:

1. Invigorates the flow of qi and blood and releases blockages
2. Disperses local qi stagnation and blood stasis, as in cases of areas of pain or visible stasis such as evidenced by the presence of spider and/or varicose veins.
3. Drain excess heat and fire from the exterior parts of the body and various internal organs.
4. Brings down yang or heat which is rising in the body (that may cause high blood pressure, migraine headaches and even lead to stroke).
5. Treats emergency conditions characterized by excess heat, epilepsy and/or mania.
6. Removes fire toxins from the body.
7. Stimulates blood production.

In summary, Hijamah has the following effects in terms of traditional medical paradigms:

Impurities:

1. Removes impurities from the blood
2. Diverts and expels toxins and harmful impurities from the vital organs

Balance of humors:

3. Removes excess blood

Heat and inflammation:

4. Draws inflammation away from the deeper organs
5. Drains excess heat and fire from the exterior parts of the body and indirectly from various internal organs.
6. Brings down yang or heat which is rising in the body (that may cause high blood pressure, migraine headaches and even lead to stroke).
7. Removes fire toxins from the body.

Circulation of blood and qi:

8. Invigorates the flow of qi and blood and releases blockages, improves blood circulation
9. Disperses local areas of qi and blood stasis, as in cases of areas of pain or visible stasis

such as evidenced by the presence of spider and/or varicose veins.

Emergency conditions:

10. Treats emergency conditions characterised by excess heat, especially where there is a mental component to the symptoms such as mania, delirium, epilepsy etc.

Stimulatory effects:

11. Stimulates blood production.
12. Assists the body's own healing abilities

Other effects:

13. Treats Sihr (black magic) and Nazr(Evil eye)

While the above effects are attributed to Hijama's uses and understanding in traditional medical paradigms, there is mounting scientific evidence to support the effects of Hijama.

Hijamah's effects based on this research will be discussed in the next section and then linked back to the effects above for a greater depth to the understanding and application of Hijamah.

Modern Medical Understanding of Hijamah

The modern medical paradigm, (which is only approximately 100 years old, beginning with the discovery of the first antibiotic in 1908), is based on different principles to traditional medicine. Though it evolved from the 4-humor theory and most drugs were and still are developed based on herbalism, modern medicine has come to define disease as based primarily on a number of distinct internal pathologies viz.:

1. Infection by a foreign organism
2. Autoimmune disorders where the body's immune system is not functioning properly
3. Genetic disorders
4. Circulatory and perfusion abnormalities (high blood pressure, ischemia etc)
5. Errors of metabolism and cell growth
6. Malfunction of glands and organs

In addition modern medicine is highly concerned with controlling and repairing:

1. Infection
2. Inflammation
3. Uncontrolled and haphazard growth of cells (as in cancer)
4. Structural deformity and injury
5. Biochemical anomalies (eg. hormonal imbalance, cholesterol markers etc.)

To a lesser extent modern medicine is also concerned with:

1. Nutrition (and states of malnutrition and nutrient deficiency)
2. Lifestyle factors

While this is not exhaustive and there are many specialties within modern medicine, they do form the foundation of medical treatment and philosophy.

Prior to 1950, bloodletting was commonly used in modern medicine for a myriad of ailments related to the above pathologies, nowadays the most common accepted use for modern bloodletting is for a hereditary iron-overload condition known as haemochromatosis. As iron builds in the patient's blood, it can have a negative impact on various areas of the body, including the heart and the joints. This can eventually lead to disease and organ failure. Bloodletting, done as phlebotomy or more often in the form of "blood donation", is applied as the main treatment for haemochromatosis, with patients having their blood taken at least once annually for life.

Hijamah however has more applications in modern medicine and the research and scientific understanding supports this, as will be demonstrated in the following pages.

Before doing so it is important to understand the difference in blood composition between blood removed via Hijamah while observing its rules and that removed by other means or methods.

Composition of the blood removed in Hijamah

The University of Damascus has conducted extensive studies on the effects of Hijamah as well as the difference in blood composition when blood is removed according to the principles of Hijamah and also against it. The following discussion is based on their research and expanded upon by myself for the benefit of the reader who may not be familiar with the medical terms and the implications of the findings.

The study first examined the nature of the blood removed where Hijamah is done according to its principles, viz:

1. For males over 20 or females after they have passed menopause,
2. In the latter part of the lunar month
3. In the spring and summer seasons,
4. In the early morning
5. In a fasting condition
6. On the upper back between the shoulder blades

When this blood is examined from the sites of incision before application of suction (so as not to alter the cell structure), the blood is found to have the following qualities:

1. The red blood cells were predominantly abnormal, including:

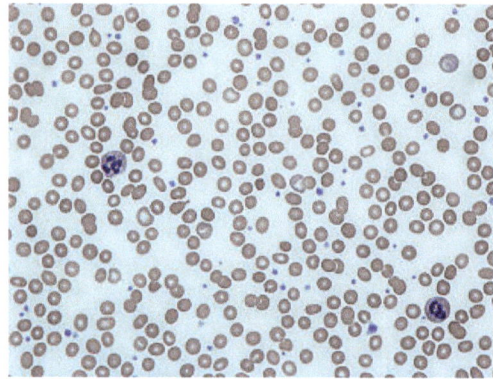

a. Hypochromic cells - these cells are normally seen in higher concentrations in patients with anemia, they appear paler than normal red blood cells. The concentration of these types of cells in healthy individuals is less than 5%. Blood removed in Hijamah however has a high number of these cells.

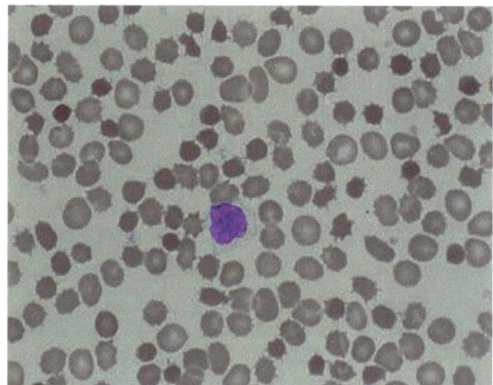

b. Burr cells - These cells are recognized by their irregular prickly shaped membrane (see above) and are regarded as aged red blood cells. Because these cells are regarded as "aged" red blood cells, they are not efficient in their function and there presence in the circulation diminishes the proper functioning of blood in the body. Hijamah blood tends to have more of these cells and when they are removed this leaves the remaining blood with a higher concentration of more efficient and younger red blood cells.

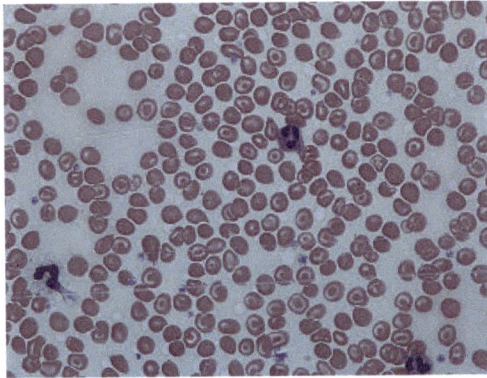

c. Target cells - (codocytes or leptocytes) have a "lump" of hemoglobinized cytoplasm within the area of normal central pallor, causing them to resemble a "bullseye" target. Target cells almost always indicate a pathological process when seen in higher than normal concentrations in regular blood samples. This is normally related to an imbalance between cholesterol and RBC ratios and may appear in association with the following conditions:

i. **Liver disease**

ii. Iron deficiency

iii. Thalassemias,

iv. Hemoglobin C diseases

v. Post-splenectomy: A major function of the spleen is the clearance of deformed, and damaged red blood cells. If splenic function is abnormal or absent because of splenectomy, abnormal RBC's will not be removed from the circulation efficiently. Therefore, increased numbers of target cells may be observed.

2. The blood sample contained less white blood cells (525 to 950 per mm3) than found in general blood samples. In adult humans, the normal range of white blood cell counts is 4500 to 11 000 per mm3. This indicates that Hijamah while removing unhealthy and aged cells does not adversely affect the concentration of healthy white blood cells which are responsible for immune functions within the blood. Amongst the WBC, it was found that lymphocytes were of greater ratio, in the region of 52% to 88%. The significance of this is not yet clear.

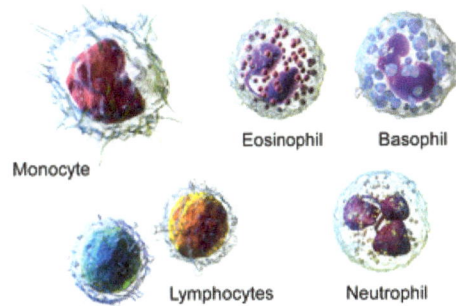

White Blood Cells

3. TIBC is significantly raised in the blood sample and indicates a very high level of transferrin present in the Hijamah blood. This may be the reason why TIBC levels are normalized in the general blood after Hijamah is performed but requires further study to elucidate its full significance. Studies have showed that high transferrin saturation in the blood is correlated with increased incidence of cancer. Hijamah therefore may be playing an important role in cancer prevention as it acts to remove a larger proportion of transferring than is present in regular blood samples or blood donation.

4. Creatinine levels are high in the Hijamah sample. This substance is a breakdown product of creatine phosphate in muscle, and normally cleared from the body by the kidneys. Hijamah seems to assist in reducing the creatinine load and thereby help "detox" the blood of this substance.

5. The plasma ratio of the Hijamah blood was approximately 20%, indicating that the process does not remove blood plasma detrimentally.

When Hijamah is done against its principles as defined above, the blood removed is of different composition and appears similar to normal venous blood, this includes when it is done on different areas of the body and out of its regular times but also in these two states that warrant special mention:

Below the recommended age

The Damascus study showed that the blood removed from younger males in Hijamah was more consistent with regular venous blood with regard to the concentration of RBCs and WBCs, the shape of RBCs as well as the levels of uric acid, cholesterol and triglycerides. The recommended age for Hijamah is above 20, though it is recommended even later than this since there are relatively less blood problems while young. This of course will depend on the individual and their particular constitution and symptoms.

On a full stomach

The study had similar findings when patients had eaten a full breakfast before having the Hijamah done. This is against the principles of Hijamah which should be done on an empty stomach since after eating the circulation is diverted to the digestive organs and away from the peripheral areas. This changes the composition of the blood removed from the Hijamah area between the shoulder blades and now it resembles normal venous blood. From anecdotal evidence many practitioners report adverse effects such as weakness, gastrointestinal upset etc when Hijamah is done on a patient who has eaten recently.

Circulatory system effects

Modern physiological understanding maintains that blood loss of less than 750ml does not have any significant physiological effect on the body and is similar to the effect of donating blood. The blood removed in the Hijamah procedure however is not the same as that lost in cases of hemorrhage due to injury or blood donation which involves phlebotomy. Studies conducted at the Damascus University in Syria observing 330 patients who received Hijamah show that upon removal of blood via performing Hijamah within its principles, the following circulatory effects were observed:

In cases of hypotension and hypertension, blood pressure returned to normal parameters - this is easily explained by the slight loss in blood volume. In the case of the individuals with hypertension the loss is not sufficient to cause vasoconstriction and results in a lower blood pressure, but in the case of hypotension, the slight loss of blood is sufficient to induce vasoconstriction and therefore increases the pressure to normal levels. There may also be other mechanisms at work involving biochemical markers. Studies confirm that Hijamah has beneficial effects on vascular compliance and degree of vascular filling and can also reduce high blood pressure in the acute setting.

(Note that the patient who is on blood pressure medication should not stop the medication after the Hijamah procedure, this may lead to a rebound effect with dangerously high blood pressure readings. It is better that the patient works with their doctor in adjusting the dosage of the medication based on the blood pressure results.)

Normalised ECG readings - In patients with ECG anomalies, the individual segments showed return to a more normal ECG pattern.

In another study published in the Chinese Journal of Physiology , the effects of Hijamah on hemodynamic parameters, arrhythmias and infarct size (IS) after myocardial ischemic reperfusion injury in male rats was studied. (Rats were induced into having a heart attack in the laboratory setting, infarct size is the size of the damaged area of heart muscle. Arrhythmias are the improper rhythm of the heart which are common with heart attacks.)

Results show that Hijamah:

- **Reduced the infarct size after injury**- this effect was most significant where hijamah was applied more than once

- **Significantly reduced Ischemic induced arrhythmias**

(This study however did not show any change in the baseline heart rate or mean arterial blood pressure.)

Effects on blood markers

ESR

The erythrocyte sedimentation rate (ESR) is the rate at which red blood cells sediment in a period of one hour. It is a common blood test, and may be an indicator of general inflammation. The ESR is increased by any cause or focus of inflammation and also in pregnancy, inflammation, anemia or rheumatoid arthritis and means that the red blood cells have a higher propensity of sticking together. It is also a diagnostic indicator for diseases such as multiple myeloma, temporal arteritis, polymyalgia rheumatica, various auto-immune diseases, systemic lupus erythematosus, rheumatoid arthritis, inflammatory bowel disease and chronic kidney diseases.

The Syrian Hijamah study showed that after Hijamah, ESR rates were lower in patients who previously had high ESR readings.

RBC count and Hb

In both cases of polycythemia where the red blood cell count is high and cases of low red blood cell count, there was a significant moderation of RBC count closer to normal values. It is already a well known treatment to use phlebotomy in patients with polycythemia but the effect of raising RBC count through bloodletting is unheard of. This can be explained by a stimulation of erythropoiesis, or red blood cell production in the body subsequent to Hijamah.
Hemoglobin levels also improved after Hijamah and may be related to the reduction of transferrin as mentioned

Thrombocytes

Thrombocyte levels were also moderated after the Hijamah procedure. In 50% of cases there was return to normal levels from either thrombocytosis or thrombocytopenia. This indicates that Hijamah has a beneficial effect for clotting problems.

Cholesterol and Triglycerides

In the Damascus study, subsequent to the Hijamah procedure, noticeable decreases in cholesterol and triglyceride levels were observed in more than 75% of patients who exhibited high levels before Hijamah. These indicators are associated with increased risk of heart disease and therefore suggest that Hijamah can reduce the risk of heart disease when done correctly.

The Iranian Society of Hijamah Research conducted further studies into this effect, the aim of the study was to determine if a there was a reduction in serum lipoproteins via Hijamah, especially LDL cholesterol, and whether it is therefore a preventive approach against atherosclerosis.

In this trial, 47 men (18 to 25 years old), without chronic disease or a history of hyperlipidemia and antihyperlipidemic drug consumption were randomly assigned into control and treated groups. Men in the treated group were subjected to Hijamah, whereas men in the control group remained untreated. The serum concentrations of lipids, collected from brachial veins, were determined at the time of Hijamah and then once a week for 3 weeks. The results showed a substantial decrease in LDL cholesterol in the treated group compared to the control. There were no significant changes in serum triglyceride between the groups however. The study concluded that Hijamah may be an effective method of reducing LDL cholesterol in men and consequently may have a preventive effect against atherosclerosis.

Glucose

Blood glucose levels were reduced in more than 80% of cases in the Damascus study. Of those who were diabetic, 92,5% experienced this reduction. Other studies also show improvement in metabolic syndrome.

Metabolic syndrome is a term used to describe the list of medical problems facing people who are obese, such as hypertension, insulin resistance and glucose intolerance. People with this condition are at risk for clots and strokes. Bloodletting can help to prevent these problems though care should be taken in bloodletting those areas with already compromised blood flow, such as the feet in diabetic patients.

Uric acid

Uric acid is a product of the metabolic breakdown of purine nucleotides in the body and its increased circulation in the blood can lead to gout. High levels are also associated with diabetes and the formation of kidney stones. In many instances, people have elevated uric acid levels for hereditary reasons, but diet may also be a factor. High intake of dietary purines (found in many meats), high fructose corn syrup, and table sugar can cause increased levels of uric acid. Serum uric acid can also be elevated due to reduced excretion by the kidneys.

The Damascus study showed improvement in uric acid levels with more than two thirds of patients undergoing Hijamah showing a decrease. This effect was more prevalent in those who had higher than normal uric acid levels to begin with. While this is a complex condition requiring other interventions including dietary and lifestyle changes as well, this shows that Hijamah can at least improve symptoms and is especially useful when done over the site of pain in the case of gout.

Liver enzymes

Liver enzymes including ALT, AST and ALP are indicative of liver damage when found in larger than normal concentrations in the blood . These enzymes are lower after the Hijamah procedure and suggest a possibility of improved liver function and health post the Hijamah procedure. Albumin levels also returned to normal in the Damascus study.

Effect of Hijamah on the organs and systems

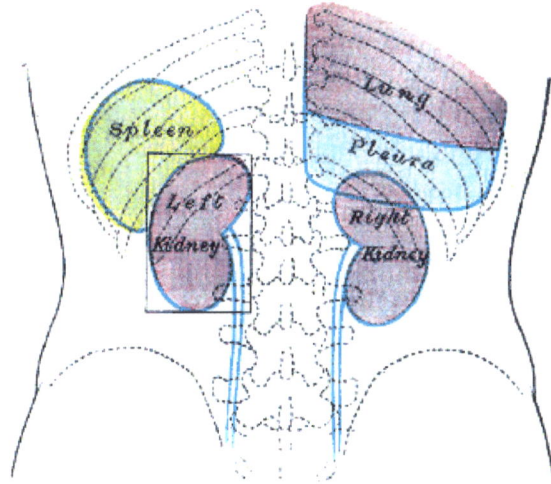

Hijamah has specific and general effects on the organs of the body and these are largely based on the indirect effects on circulation and altering of the blood composition described above. There are some direct effects however that relate to the area being bled and its connection with the particular organ

Spleen

The spleen is an organ in the body that acts as a blood filter—It removes old red blood cells and holds a reserve of blood in case of massive blood loss. It also recycles iron and has an important role in the function of the immune system. Disorders of the spleen include splenomegaly, where the spleen is enlarged for various reasons, such as cancer, specifically blood-based leukemias, and asplenia, where the spleen is not present or functions abnormally.

From the results of the composition of Hijamah blood, it is clear that Hijamah can reduce the load on the spleen by assisting in its function of removing aged blood cells and thereby assist with splenomegaly where it is due to congestion of the spleen due to inability to process large amounts of damaged or old RBCs. Hijamah is also necessary where the spleen has been removed.

Liver

The liver is a vital organ that has a wide range of functions in the human body, including detoxification, protein synthesis and production of biochemicals necessary for digestion. This organ plays a major role in metabolism and has a number of essential functions in the body, including glycogen storage, decomposition of red blood cells, plasma protein synthesis, hormone production, and detoxification. Because of its location and various functions, the liver is prone to many diseases such as

1. Infections such as hepatitis
2. Alcohol damage,
3. Fatty liver
4. Cirrhosis
5. Cancer
6. Drug damage

Many diseases of the liver are accompanied by jaundice caused by increased levels of bilirubin in the system. The bilirubin results from the breakup of the hemoglobin of dead red blood cells; normally, the liver removes bilirubin from the blood and excretes it through bile.

Because the liver can easily become overworked Hijamah has an effect on the liver similar to its effect on the spleen in that it reduces the work required by the liver in detoxifying the body and removing waste products. Hijamah therefore may assist in all the above liver diseases and also the resulting jaundice that may occur.

Kidneys

The effect on the kidneys is similar to that on the spleen. Hijamah assists the kidneys filtration function and lessens its load by removing impurities directly from the blood. After the procedure there is also heightened activity by the kidney in releasing erythropoietin which stimulates production of new red blood cells.

Nervous system

Anecdotal evidence shows that Hijamah is useful for both restoring proper blood flow to the brain (in cases of ischaemia) as well as reducing pressure in the brain when it is high. Hijamah may therefore be useful in the prevention and treatment of stroke, and it is also noted for its ability to improve memory and focus as reported by those who have had it done.

Effect of Hijamah on particular diseases

A number of studies have been conducted on the effect of Hijamah on particular illnesses and conditions. Exact treatment details on each disease are left for my practitioner level book but some research studies and reviews are described here for the benefit of the patient.

General research

1. The US Public Library of Science published a review in 2012 of all studies that examined the efficacy of cupping therapy. Only studies with randomized control trials were included in their analysis. What they were able to conclude after reviewing 135 experiments was that a) cupping therapy does not yield any serious adverse side effects, and b) cupping therapy was significantly better at improving patients' health when combined with other treatments compared to the other treatments alone. Combined therapy yielded more cured patients in these studies, especially those afflicted with shingles, facial paralysis (as with Bell's Palsy), acne, and spondylosis (or osteoarthritis of the neck)[6]

2. A systematic review published in BMC Complementary and Alternative Medicine in 2010 concluded that the majority of studies show potential benefit for pain conditions, herpes zoster and a number of other diseases.[7]

These studies confirm that Hijamah does not have adverse effects when done properly and more importantly confirms that it is indeed therapeutic in nature.

Diabetes

Recent studies conducted by Unani Practitioners in India[8] show that when Hijamah is combined with other therapies for Diabetes Mellitus, effectiveness of the therapy is increased in the treatment group. Hijamah was administered every month on the 17th day of the lunar calendar in keeping with the "Hijamah in Strength" principles. Symptoms such as polydipsia, polyphagia and polyuria were more improved in the treatment versus control group. The treatment group also showed improvement in wound healing, and lower blood glucose and cholesterol levels.

This study confirms the findings of the Damascus study showing that blood glucose (and cholesterol) levels are improved with Hijamah and therefore should be combined with regular therapies for the treatment of Diabetes Mellitus. This of course should be done in keeping with the principles and having Hijamah every month should only be done if the climate is conducive to it. Excessive amounts of blood should not be removed if it is a monthly practice.

Pain

Hijamah is very effective for pain conditions and is probably the most common indication for Hijamah in the clinic setting. Anecdotal evidence suggests all types of pain disorders are well treated by Hijamah with the practitioner using different points on the body depending on the presenting signs and symptoms. There are a number of studies that support this:

In a Korean study[9] Hijamah was found to be superior than heat packs in improving neck pain, function and discomfort in cases of neck pain due to computer work.

A few studies[10,11], also show that Hijamah is better than regular therapies in the treatment of lower back pain. In these studies Hijamah was associated with clinically significant improvement post treatment and at 3-month follow-up. The group who received Hijamah had significantly lower levels of pain intensity, pain-related disability and medication use than the control group.

Headaches are also well treated by Hijamah[12]. In one study, 70 patients with chronic tension or migraine headache were treated with Hijamah. Three primary outcome measures were considered at the baseline and 3 months following treatment: headache severity, days of headache per month, and use of medication. The results of the study showed that, compared to the baseline, headache severity decreased by 66% following Hijamah treatment. Treated patients also experienced the 12.6 fewer days of headache per month and had less reliance on pain medication. Hijamah therefore has clinically relevant benefits for patients with headache.

Shingles pain is another area where research has verified the effects of Hijamah. In a review[13] of 8 randomised controlled trials to evaluate the therapeutic effect of Hijamah for herpes zoster, the studies showed that Hijamah was better than medication for Herpes Zoster, in terms of the number of completely cured patients, the number of patients with improved symptoms, and the incidence rate of post-herpetic neuralgia (pain). The combination of Hijamah with medication was significantly better than medication alone.

Researchers also investigated the effect of Hijamah on Carpal Tunnel Syndrome , 52 patients with neurologically confirmed CTS were randomly assigned to either a treatment group which received Hijamah or a control group that had an application of a heat pack. Hijamah patients were treated with a single application of wet cupping, and control patients with a single local application of heat within the region overlying the trapezius muscle. Patients were followed up on day 7 after treatment. The primary outcome, severity of CTS symptoms (VAS), had greater reduction in the Hijamah group than in the control group, other aspects were also more improved in the Hijamah group, including neck pain, functional disability and physical quality of life. The treatment was safe and well tolerated. The researchers concluded that Hijamah may be effective in relieving the pain and other symptoms related to Carpal Tunnel Syndrome.

Other diseases

Though Hijamah enjoys such wide and frequent use, it remains more popular in countries that do not regularly publish research studies in english accessible journals, as a result research is still sparse on other conditions though anecdotal evidence and my own personal experience suggest that Hijamah is also effective, especially when combined with other therapies for the following illnesses:

- Gynecological disorders, including amenorrhea, infertility, endometriosis etc
- Dermatological (skin) disorders, including eczema, dermatitis, acne
- Neurological disorders including stroke, spinal cord injury, certain types of epilepsy etc
- Gastrointestinal disorders, especially those characterised by inflammation, including gastritis, nausea and vomiting, some infectious conditions etc

A novel scientific theory explaining the medical effects of Hijamah was proposed by Salah Mohamed El Sayed from the Department of Medical Biochemistry of the Suhag university in Egypt. This theory, termed Taiba theory, described in the May 2013 edition of the journal Alternative and Integrated Medicine is currently the most accurate scientific explanation of Hijamah's curative properties.

Salah named this theory "Taibah" theory after the city of the Nabi ﷺ, Madinah Munawwara in present day Saudi Arabia. Taibah is one of the names of this peaceful and blessed city and it means "clean", "pure" or "excellent". It also refers the ability of Madinah to purify its inhabitants and because it removes from it those that are impure and of ill-intention.

In summary, Taibah theory explains that *Hijamah is a minor surgical excretory procedure and its effect is similar to the mechanism of excretory function via glomerular filtration of the kidney, as well as abscess drainage, by which pathological (disease causing) substances are removed from the body.* This theory will be described in more detail below as presented by Salah in his paper.

There are a few stages in the Hijamah procedure; first a cup is applied with suction before any piercing of the skin is performed. The cup is then removed after which the skin is pierced and the cup reapplied in order to draw blood from the resulting incisions.

1. When negative pressure is applied to the skin surface the first time a cup (or horn) is applied, the skin surface is lifted up into the cup due to its viscoelastic nature. The local pressure around the capillaries present inside this pocket lifted into the cup decreases and causes increased capillary filtration and thereby collection of filtered fluids which include causative pathogenic substances (CPS), old and damaged red blood cells, in addition to lymph and interstitial fluid in the interstitial space of this pocket. Chemical substances, inflammatory mediators and nociceptive substances released bathe the nerve endings present in the pocket resulting in analgesia, while any tissue adhesions are broken adding to the pain relieving effect of Hijamah.

2. When the cups are removed, a dramatic local increase in blood flow occurs, termed reactive hyperemia.

3. At the next stage incisions are made, before the cup is reapplied. The incisions allow removal of the CPS and collected fluids mentioned above and prevent their reabsorption into the venous system. It also causes release of endogenous opioids that add to the analgesic effect.

4. The second application of the cup and resultant negative pressure is transmitted through the incisions and creates a pressure gradient that causes excretion of the collected fluids that contains the CPS into the cup. Aged blood cellular fragments, and molecules and particles

smaller than the capillary pore sizes selectively pass through the capillary pores under the negative pressure effect, while intact blood cells (larger than the size of pores and fenestrae of skin capillaries) do not. This explains the preponderance of unhealthy RBC's in Hijamah blood.

The negative pressure suction and also release of nitric oxide, helps to dilate local blood capillaries.

Salah explains this improves microcirculation, increases capillary permeability, increases drainage of excess fluids, increases lymph clearance and flow, decreases absorption at the venous end of capillaries, increases fluid filtration at both arterial and venous capillary ends, and increases fluid excretion (filtered fluids and interstitial fluids) which acts to treat blood congestion, improve blood and lymphatic capillary circulation and resolve tissue swelling (due to removal of CPS, noxious substances, prostaglandins and inflammatory mediators).

The positive effects of this include:

1. Improving oxygen supply,
2. Enhancing tissue perfusion and cellular metabolism
3. Preserving underlying tissue structure
4. Modulating angiogenesis
5. Relieving muscle spasm
6. Restoring balance of the neuro-endocrine system
7. Improving neurotransmission
8. Exerting pharmacological potentiation
9. Restoring physiological homeostasis.

Salah advises that Hijamah should be done whenever excess CPS or fluids are to be excreted. This can be determined either by applying Hijamah in strength for the person whose constitution allows it or by using the principles of Hijamah in illness by assessing the patient through differential diagnosis.

Who should practice Hijamah

Hijamah is regarded as an invasive medical procedure and more importantly is such a procedure where the skin is pierced and there is subsequent handling of body fluids. Any such procedure in medicine presents with a large number of risks when compared to procedures where the skin is not pierced and there is no handling of body fluids.

In recent years there has been a proliferation of dangerous infections that are transmitted easily through blood and body fluids. These include HIV, Hepatitis B, Hepatitis C and Viral Hemorrhagic Fever. Since it is difficult to determine what infectious pathogens any given blood contains, and some blood-borne diseases are lethal, standard medical practice regards all blood (and any body fluid) as potentially infectious.

There are many cases where Hijamah has resulted in infection with the HIV and Hepatitis viruses, at least one documented HIV infection has occurred in Saudi Arabia and two documented cases reported in Iranian studies. *(The majority of cases go undocumented as the patients may not be aware that they have been infected and/or practitioners neglect to report adverse effects for fear of prosecution)*

Other risks of Hijamah are also inherent in terms of dealing with the effects of excessive blood loss *(which may occur due to hereditary disease or medication the patient is taking)*, incorrect piercing of the skin and subsequent damage to nerves or blood vessels, all of which can potentially be fatal for the patient. Improper handling and disposal of body fluids and sharps is also a common occurrence by those practicing Hijamah without proper training and presents a serious risk of spread of infection to other members of the community.

For this reason it is the opinion of many Ulama that the Hajjaam must be an individual who has had biomedical training, either a medical doctor or a qualified and registered practitioner of complementary medicine, or at least an individual who has received specific training in Hijamah and has also received with it training in human anatomy, physiology, general pathology, clinical medicine, clinical diagnostics, differential diagnosis, pharmacological interactions and how to properly handle body fluids and prevent infections.

Most countries have a register of individuals who are qualified to practice medicine, whether conventional or complementary, and amongst these there are those who have learnt and practice Hijamah. In some countries like the UK there are specific registers for practitioners of Hijamah and such individuals have received training in the safe application of the procedure. These should be the individuals who are first sought for having Hijamah done and if one is interested in practicing Hijamah then one should endeavor to learn it properly with its necessary biomedical prerequisites in order to gain such formal qualification and registration.

Individuals who practice Hijamah without the necessary qualifications are opening themselves up to prosecution by the law in their country should anything go wrong whether it be their own carelessness or by chance. Medical malpractice litigation is becoming more and more common and an unregistered practitioner has no support in such a case from any health council or registration body.

In the US the regulations regarding Hijamah only allow the following licensed professionals to practice;

- Physicians
- Physicians Assistants (PA)
- Advanced Practitioner Registered Nurse (APRN)
- Licensed Acupincturist (LAc)
- Phlebotomists-Only allowed to draw blood in lab setting.
- Paramedics-Allowed to draw blood or do incisions in emergency situations only.

Of course there are some countries where the law is not strict about such matters, but the practitioner will have to live with the consequences of their lack of knowledge and experience in medical matters should something go wrong while practicing Hijamah.

Many believe that Hijamah is exclusively an Islaamic practice and therefore it should be legalised for any Muslim to practice it. This is erroneous since Hijamah is a medical practice that was already present before the coming of the Nabi ﷺ and was encouraged by the Nabi ﷺ, it is not specific to any particular religion or culture but rather it is a treatment for the entire world. Unlike the use of honey and black seed, Hijamah is a medical procedure and because in Islaam we are taught to take precaution and not engage in anything that can cause harm to us both spiritually and physically, one should seek out an expert in Hijamah, who also has the necessary biomedical qualifications for the procedure.

General contraindications and precautions

As is discussed above, Hijamah is not without its risks, and it is not for everybody to undertake. The Hajjaam must see that the patient is fit for Hijamah and must know how to adapt the procedure based on the constitution of the patient and their current state of health. This is also borne out by the hadith:

Jabir bin Abdullaah (RA) relates that he heard Rasulullaah ﷺ saying: "If there is any good in your treatments it is in the blade of the Hajjaam, a drink of honey or branding by fire (cauterisation/moxibustion), whichever suits the ailment, and I do not like to be cauterized" *(Bukhari & Muslim)*

This hadith infers that one must know if Hijamah is the best treatment for the patient, or another treatment would be more suitable. It is interesting to note that in this same hadith the 3 main principles of treatment are referred to, viz, supplementing (with honey), draining heat (by Hijamah) and treating cold and stasis (with fire).

In order to know if Hijamah will suit the patient the Hajjaam must first know the contraindications and precautions for practicing Hijamah. Contraindications being those conditions if present, in which Hijamah should not be done and precautions being those in which it is not prohibited, but caution should be observed, especially in terms of how much blood is removed.

Excessive perspiration

"Do not bleed the one who is sweating, do not sweat the one who is bleeding"

The first rule of preventing adverse effects of Hijamah is not to perform the procedure for a person who is suffering from excessive perspiration. In traditional medicine this is understood as a weakness of the body in its ability to hold the pores closed, which therefore results in excessive and easy perspiration. (This should not be confused with night sweats which are a different phenomenon mostly due to heat forcing the pores open at night.)

A person who suffers from easy and excessive sweating is already suffering from a loss of body fluids and bleeding such a person will only aggravate this condition. They will also tend to bleed more easily and may exhibit excessive and uncontrolled blood loss should Hijamah be performed. Excessive sweating, or hyperhidrosis, can be a warning sign of thyroid problems, diabetes or infection. It is also more common in people who are overweight or out of shape. Such an individual is not normally suffering from an "excess heat" type of condition where Hijamah is indicated.

The second part of this precaution, viz. do not sweat the one who is one bleeding, means that medication which is used to cause sweating (diaphoretics) should not be used in a person who is bleeding (as it will increase blood loss unnecessarily).

Hemophilia

Hemophilia is a genetic disorder that impairs the body's ability to control blood clotting or coagulation, which is used to stop bleeding when a blood vessel is broken, or to heal the incision that is created by the Hajjaam. It is more common in males than females and is characterized by lower blood plasma clotting factor levels of the coagulation factors needed for a normal clotting process. Thus when a blood vessel is injured, a temporary scab does form, but the missing coagulation factors prevent fibrin formation, which is necessary to maintain the blood clot. A hemophiliac does not bleed more intensely than a person without it, but can bleed for a much longer time. In severe hemophiliacs even a minor incision from Hijamah can result in blood loss lasting days or weeks, or even never healing completely. For this reason it is not recommended to perform Hijamah on a hemophiliac, unless it is in association with their medical practitioner who understands the severity and nature of the patients hemophilia and regards Hijamah as safe for the patient.

The Hajjaam should take a proper history of the patient in order to determine if the patient is a hemophiliac.

Anticoagulant drugs

If a patient is on medication, the Hajjaam must determine whether it is safe to continue with Hijamah and that the medication will not cause excessive and potentially uncontrollable bleeding or other adverse effects.

Amongst these medications the most dangerous are anticoagulant medicines. Anticoagulants are medicines that prevent the blood from clotting as quickly or as effectively as normal. Some people call anticoagulants blood thinners. However, the blood is not actually made any thinner - it just does not clot so easily whilst you take an anticoagulant.

Anticoagulants are commonly used to treat and prevent blood clots that may occur in your blood vessels. Blood clots can block an artery or a vein. A blocked artery stops blood and oxygen from getting to a part of your body (for example, to a part of the heart, brain or lungs). The tissue supplied by a blocked artery becomes damaged, or dies, and this results in serious problems such as a stroke or heart attack. A blood clot in a large vein, such as a deep vein thrombosis (a clot in the leg vein), can lead to serious problems such as a pulmonary embolism (a clot that travels from the leg vein to the lungs).

Patients on anticoagulant medication may exhibit excessive blood loss after Hijamah

which in some cases can be fatal. The most common anticoagulants include warfarin and heparin, however these may go by different brand names and for this reason a Hajjaam should be familiar with basic pharmacology and be able to recognize anticoagulant use in prospective Hijamah patients. If you are using anticoagulants you should consult with your doctor before having Hijamah done.

If you are not sure whether you are using anticoagulant medication you can check your medication against this list of common names for anticoagulant medication, the list is not exhaustive and ideally your Hajjaam should have the knowledge and training to identify if you are using an anticoagulant or not:

Warfarin	Coumadin, Jantoven, Marevan, Lawarin, Waran, Warfant
Dabigatran	Pradaxa
Acenocoumarol	G 23350, Nicoumalone, Nicumalon
Phenindione	Dindevan, Fenindion, Phenylin-Zdorovye, Soluthrombine
Rivaroxaban	Xarelto

Note: Aspirin also has an effect of preventing clots by preventing platelets sticking together. However, it is classed as an antiplatelet agent rather than an anticoagulant.

Anemia

Anemia is a common condition in which the blood lacks adequate healthy red blood cells. Red blood cells carry oxygen to the body's tissues. Iron deficiency anemia is due to insufficient iron. Without enough iron, the body cannot produce enough hemoglobin, a substance in red blood cells that enables them to carry oxygen. As a result, iron deficiency anemia may leave an individual tired and short of breath.

A number of recent studies , are showing a link between excessive and unnecessary bloodletting and iron deficiency anemia, some even as severe as resulting in cardiomyopathy which is only seen in chronic severe iron deficiency anaemia.

For this reason care should be taken not to cause this type of anemia through Hijamah. This will most often occur when women who are menstruating normally receive Hijamah without a serious reason, or when Hijamah is practiced too often and/or too much blood is removed.

For the healthy person not living in a very hot climate, to have Hijamah once a year in the hot season is sufficient, provided the person exhibits signs of a healthy constitution and does not already suffer from anemia. If so, then it should be administered in a "low dose" only once every few years so as to encourage haematopoiesis. (For a women who is menstruating general Hijamah is not needed except where the woman is suffering from an abundance of blood as sometimes happens in the arab regions.)

Pregnancy

During pregnancy there is a tremendous demand by the baby for nourishment which is provided by means of the mothers blood. For this reason the woman's appetite grows tremendously due to the increased production of blood in her body. This is the system that Allaah ﷻ has created to provide for the child in the womb of the mother. The heat of the body is also concentrated internally during the pregnancy period which leaves the outer parts relatively cold and lacking in blood. The normal menstrual cycle also ceases, which in traditional medicine is seen as a sign that there is no need for the woman to lose blood in this period. As a result, if Hijamah is applied in such a stage then great harm is done to the body and to the developing baby, this can easily result in miscarriage.

It is shocking to me when I hear that women who are pregnant are having Hijamah done, and on more than one occasion I have come to know that this has resulted in miscarriage. The irresponsible Hajjaam then hides behind the claim of "taqdeer" when in fact this is medical malpractice and they will be held responsible in the court of Allaah ﷻ for not adhering to basic medical guidelines in respect of care during pregnancy.

Pregnancy is a clear contraindication for Hijamah, it should not be done or even considered during pregnancy and should a Hajjaam either due to ignorance or pursuit of money cause a miscarriage then the Hajjaam is to blame and in m y opinion should be charged with a crime by the legal system prevailing in that country.

Wound healing disorders

When performing Hijamah incisions are made in the skin to release blood. Normally these heal within a short period and leave minimal scarring (especially when a post Hijamah blood and healing herbal formula and/or low level laser therapy is applied afterward).

In some conditions however, the body's ability to heal and repair the incision is impaired, and results in either a longer healing time, no healing at all or excessive scarring and keloid formation.
Example of Keloid formed after an operation due to a motorcycle accident

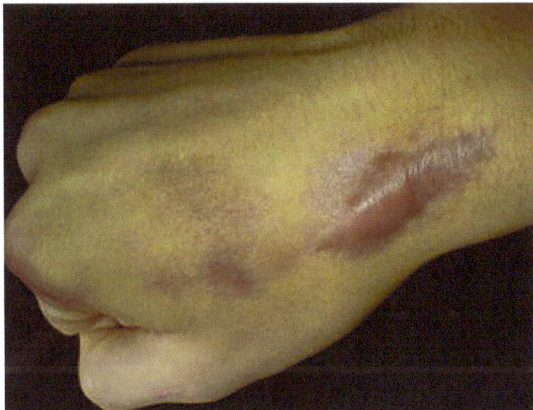

Keloids are thickened scars due to excessive synthesis of collagen after an acute injury, which can include the incision, required for Hijamah. Hypertrophic scarring and keloids most frequently arise in young adults and are particularly prevalent in dark-skinned individuals. They are equally common in males and females. These scars may also itch and/or be painful to touch. They are firm or hard, skin-coloured to bright red, smooth, elevated nodules and may have claw-like extensions far beyond the original wound.

They are particularly frequently seen on earlobes, shoulders, upper back and anterior chest. Hijamah should be avoided in individuals who have a history of easily developing keloids and hypertrophic scarring. (This is not a contraindication but rather a precaution as we have experienced less occurrence of keloids if the patient is exposed to low level laser therapy after the procedure)

Healing of the incisions can also be impaired by other factors that slow down or prevent complete healing and include issues such as the lack of growth factors, the presence of edema, poor blood flow, infection, hypoxia, arterial or venous insufficiency and neuropathy.

Other systemic causes of impaired wound healing include metabolic disease, diabetes mellitus, the patients nutritional state, a history of smoking or drug use, exposure to radiation, aging, immune disorders, and abnormal collagen syndromes. A thorough history will reveal if the patient may have wound healing problems.

Diabetes deserves special mention as it is a common disorder and when present gives rise to a high risk of major complications in the Hijamah incision, including infection and cellulitis and can even lead to amputation when performed on the extremities.
Vascular, neuropathic, immune function, and biochemical abnormalities in diabetes each contribute to delayed healing. Even careful wound care in a patient with excellent glucose control may fail and result in these adverse

effects. Special care should therefore be taken in diabetic patients in order to determine whether Hijamah is appropriate for the patient and if so, it should be done only in those areas and in a way that will not risk poor wound healing, subsequent infection and other adverse effects.

Who should have Hijamah done

In the hadith related by Jabir ibn Abdullaah (RA), the Nabi ﷺ, said: توافق الداء meaning "whichever fits the ailment", in these 2 words the entire field of differential diagnosis and differential treatment was proven and emphasised. In this particular hadith the Nabi of Allaah ﷺ said this in respect of the 3 treatments of honey, hijamah and cauterisation.

This indicates that albeit established that the contraindications are not present and the precautions are observed, Hijamah may not be the appropriate treatment for the patient.

In order to determine if Hijamah fits the patient and their ailment the Hajjaam should possess some basic skills of differential diagnosis. This includes both western and traditional medicine diagnostic skills in order to determine two essential aspects, viz:

- The constitution or body type of the patient
- The root syndrome of the illness

Being able to determine these two aspects will guide the Hajjaam as to whether Hijamah fits the ailment or not.

Constitutions or body types

Hippocrates said that: "It is more important to know what sort of person has a disease, than to know what sort of a disease a person has."

This principle has all but completely departed from the practice of modern medicine but still remains an integral part of the practice of traditional medicine like Unani-Tibb and TCM. It is perhaps the most important criteria in both the identification of the nature of the disease as well as the selection of a treatment method.
Understanding the type of person, their temperament as well as their lifestyle, social and environmental influences and history can make the difference between a successful resolution of the presenting illness and a litany of inaccurate diagnoses and ineffective treatments.

Recognising the body types is not difficult to master. There are 4 primary constitutions or body types within the Unani philosophy and 5 within the Traditional Chinese Medicine philosophy. These can be combined into 5 main body types for the purposes of determining the suitability of Hijamah. They are as follows:

Fire constitution (Hot and Moist - Sanguinous)

They have a strong circulatory system and manifest with red facial hues. These individuals have a hotter temperament, their build is large with more muscle, the skin is warmer, their complexion is reddish in colour and glowing, and the veins are prominent.

They usually have broad paravertebral muscles and well-proportioned shoulders, upper back and thighs. Their head is smaller and somewhat pointed, with a pointed chin, small hands and feet and usually curly hair, often these individuals may have an early receding hairline.

They suffer from excessive thirst and are uncomfortable in the hot season. They tend to wear less clothing than others do and will sleep with the windows open. They may also be short in stature (dynamite in a small package) and have an "explosive" personality and tend to excessive laughter, they are persuasive, sociable, outgoing, talkative, all embracing, affectionate, expansive, generous, intuitive, warm and bright.

Fire personalities are trusting, open minded, social, and fond of beauty.

They are spontaneous and often funny.

Potential disorders they may suffer from include insomnia, arrhythmias, paranoia, restlessness, palpitations, nervous exhaustion, anxiety, agitation.

Wood constitution - (Hot and Dry - Bilious)

They have softer skin, more fat, medium to muscular body with prominent veins. They are resourceful, outspoken, and may be short-tempered.

Other words that describe them may include forceful, determined, bold, decisive, clear, tendency to overdo, over direct, over perform.

They also have small and shapely hands and feet, broad shoulders and a straight flat back. By nature these individuals enjoy the spring and summer seasons and tend to dislike autumn and winter, as their constitution leaves them more vulnerable to pathogenic invasion and disease during these seasons. They have strong sinews and tendons and tend to manifest with green bluish facial hues.

Wood constitutions tend to be kind, merciful, creative, and free in self-expression.

They can also manifest stubbornness, dominance and may have issues with anger, excessive aggressiveness and are almost always overachievers. When sick they can be unassertive, unsure of themselves and their role in life.

They may experience difficulties in expressing themselves, and have weak boundaries, and display timidity and self-doubt.

Potential disorders include blood glucose issues, PMS, muscle pains, allergies and hayfever, depressive episodes, epilepsy, intolerance, impatience, vascular or migraine headaches, They may also suffer from diarrhea and frequent indigestion.

Metal constitution (Cold and Dry - Melancholic)

Their skin is dry and rough, they are more slender than the average, appear thin and bony and dont put on weight easily even though they may have a voracious appetite, they do not tolerate dry foods. They like moist things, hot water and thin oils are readily absorbed by their skin. The complexion is sometimes described as greyish, sooty or otherwise they appear white and pale but not shiny, they tend to be thoughtful, logical, analytical, and are perfectionists. Other words that describe them include self restraint, methodical, efficient, and disciplined, lives according to principle, sense of symmetry, logical mind, purity of ideals.

Potential disorders include frequent Infections, chronic cough, COPD, sinus infections, dry skin, hair, skin disorders, stiff joints and muscles, shallow breathing, poor circulation.

Water constitution (Cold and Moist - Phlegmatic)

These individuals are often overweight and their skin feels cold to the touch. They have thin hair, a whitish shiny complexion, and laxity in the joints. In cold weather they become pale, leaden colored and have small veins. Their digestion is sluggish and often suffers from constipation. They tend to have a large round face, head and body, long upper back, large hips and may have uneven physical proportions.

They tend to be calm, accommodating, patient and good listeners.

Potential disorders include edema, urinary infections, impotence and infertility, low back weakness and pain, weak knees, deterioration of teeth, loss of libido.

Earth constitution

These individuals tend to have somewhat larger bodies and over proportioned head and abdomen, strong thighs, round face and wide jaw line. Their limbs are well proportioned and they often carry excess "flesh".

Balanced Earth personalities are predisposed to quiet peaceful lives unconcerned with wealth and fame. They are always at peace, calm and generous, forgiving and sincere. In life they are analytical, practical and logical with strong adaptability to changing circumstances.

Earth constitutions can develop digestive and gastrointestinal tract illnesses as these organs can get injured with excessive worrying and over thinking.

Qualities that describe an earth constitution include being practical, down-to-earth, intelligent, anticipating, meeting needs of the family, kind, supportive, pliant, reliable. They can sometimes however become too pushy and possessive.

Potential disorders include weight difficulties, obsessions, worry, self-doubt, digestive disturbances, low energy, cold limbs, food allergies, weak muscles, and unrealistic expectations, meddling, overprotective.

Constitutions suited to Hijamah

Of these only the Fire, Wood and to a lesser extent Earth constitutions are suited to regular Hijamah. These constitutions display an excess of either (liver/heart) heat and blood in the case of the fire type, (liver) heat and stagnation in the case of the wood type, or stagnation and (stomach) heat in the case of the Earth type. They therefore benefit tremendously from Hijamah done as a general health preservation modality.

For the other constitutions, Hijamah is not generally indicated and if done must be done keeping in mind the principles of Hijamah done in illness. Too much blood must also not be removed as these individuals are already either deficient in blood (metal type) or deficient in heat (water type). There are times however when Hijamah applied in specific areas and for specific illnesses can be beneficial. This is described in further detail below:

8 patterns of illness

One method of understanding the basic nature of an illness is to assess the ailment in terms of the "8 patterns". These are in fact 4 sets of opposing concepts viz.:

Hot / Cold
Internal / External
Excess / Deficiency
Yin / Yang

When determining if an illness is suited to treatment by Hijamah we are mostly concerned with 2 of these sets, viz. hot/cold and excess/deficiency.
There are a number of ways to determine and differentiate how the ailment relates to

these concepts such as through asking about the presenting symptoms, as well as looking at the tongue and feeling the pulse.

Pulse and tongue diagnosis are specialist fields that require practical training and therefore full detail is not provided on these aspects of diagnosis. Briefly, for Hijamah to be suitable for the ailment, the pulse should be rapid, floating or surging, not slow, deep or weak. it also should not be floating or hollow in the center. (For practitioners who want to explore the fascinating field of pulse diagnosis in detail I suggest signing up for my next course on pulse diagnosis here: www.pulsediagnosiscourse.com)

Asking about the symptoms in order to determine the nature of the illness is a method that is accessible to most and can provide enough information in the majority of cases to come to a diagnosis vis. a vie the pattern of illness.

When determining heat we differentiate between excess heat or deficient heat.

Excess heat has the following characteristics:

Main Signs: Fever (sometimes), thirst, red face, red eyes, constipation. Urine is scanty and dark.

Pulse: Rapid and Full

Tongue: Red with a yellow coating

The following are some general signs of an Excess Heat pattern though the exact symptoms depend on the organ(s) affected.

- Raised, red skin eruption that feels hot e.g. acute urticaria
- Any burning painful sensation e.g. urine or stomach pain
- Loss of blood with large quantities of bright red blood indicates Heat in the Blood
- Extreme mental restlessness/manic behavior (Heat in the Heart)
- Thick, yellow, sticky, malodorous secretions/excretions

Excess Heat patterns are caused by excess of energy and blood in the body and individuals presenting with this type of pattern will respond very well to Hijamah.

Deficient heat has the following characteristics:

Main Signs: Afternoon fever or feeling of heat in afternoon, dry mouth, dry throat at night, night sweats, fever in 5 hearts, dry stools, scanty-dark urine, mental restlessness and fidgeting, vague anxiety. (More specific signs depend on Organ involved)

Pulse: Floating-Empty and Rapid or Thin and Rapid

Tongue: Red, in severe cases peeled. No Coating.

Other signs that may be present:

- Deficiency heat affecting the Lung - Malar flush, dry cough.
- Deficiency heat affecting the Liver - Headaches, dry eyes, irritability.

- Deficiency heat affecting the Heart - palpitations, insomnia and feelings of restlessness.
- Deficiency heat can be caused by many factors, stress being a major one.
- Excessive sexual indulgence, overwork, smoking, alcohol and drug abuse, all deplete the fluids and give rise to this type of heat as well.
- Long-standing emotional distress can also cause this pattern.

Such patients are suited to Hijamah but only with small quantities of blood removed. If the patient is suffering from excessive sweating then Hijamah is contraindicated.

Circulation issues

Irrespective of the constitution, circulation problems are well treated by Hijamah provided that the area affected is treated directly. In order to determine if the circulation is affected in a particular area of the body, the practitioner will have to take a thorough history and examine the area. Though full detail is beyond the scope of this book and must be learned through a course in clinical diagnostic skills in addition to other subjects, there are some signs that indicate poor circulation, viz:

- There are feels cold to the touch when compared to other areas
- There are prominent spider veins which appear purplish in nature.
- The patient experiences pain of a sharp and stabbing nature in the area
- There are purple spots on the tongue corresponding with the affected body area.

In these cases Hijamah may be beneficial though some special techniques must be employed such as bleeding of the spider veins etc.

Geographical considerations

Modern medicine has not fully understood the effect of the climate on the health of individuals, yet traditional and complementary medical systems place tremendous emphasis on the climate, season and prevailing weather in the geographical area that a person resides in. Hakims are famous for recommending some patients move to another town or city that had a more favorable climate as the only method of treatment for the patients ailment.

Similarly, the climate and weather must be taken into account when determining the suitability of Hijamah as is also borne out by this hadith:

*Anas ibn Maalik (RA) reported that the Rasul ﷺ said, "**When the weather becomes extremely hot, seek aid in Hijamah**. Do not allow your blood to rage (boil) such that it kills you." [Reported by Hakim in his 'Mustadrak' and he authenticated it and Imam ad-Dhahabi agreed (4/212)].*

From this we learn that Hijamah is suited to the hot climate, and this is corroborated by other Ahadeeth as well. If the patient lives in a region where the climate is normally hot, then Hijamah is probably suited to the patient. If the patient lives in a region where it is always cold, then care should be taken even if the patient displays the correct constitution for Hijamah. Every patient's condition will be different and it is up to the skilled and experienced Hajjaam to determine the weight of the climate, season and prevailing weather on the suitability of Hijamah.

One may find that the season is correct, the dates are correct, the patient is suited to Hijamah but the particular weather on that day is cold and rainy. I would normally avoid doing Hijamah on such a day and postpone it to another day if it were a general Hijamah.

In the commentary on the books of Ahadeeth, Ulama have also written the following which must be considered:

"The saying of Sayyidina Rasulullaah ﷺ that cupping is the best medicine is very true. By this he was addressing the youth of the Haramayn, and also the inhabitants of the countries where the climate is hot, because their blood becomes thin, it remains more on the surface of the body and the climate of the country brings it even more closer to the surface."

The condition of the person having Hijamah

If Hijamah has been deemed suitable the patient must ensure to prepare themselves and be in the appropriate condition for the procedure. This is evident from a number of Ahadeeth such as the following:

*Ibn Umar (RA) reported that the Rasul ﷺ said, "**Hijamah on an empty stomach is best**. In it is a cure and a blessing..." [Saheeh Sunan ibn Maajah (3487)].*

Ibn Umar (RA) reported that the Rasul ﷺ said, "Hijamah on an empty stomach is best. In it is a cure and a blessing. **It improves the intellect and the memory**..." [Saheeh Sunan ibn Maajah (3487)].*

This is the most important condition, i.e. the patient should have an empty stomach.

The reason for this, especially in the case of Hijamah in strength, is because during the night, the toxins and impurities in the blood accumulate in the regions where Hijamah is done and remain there until a person eats. When a meal is taken blood is redirected to the digestive organs to enable the process of digestion and absorption.

The toxins and impurities are therefore recirculated throughout the body instead of being concentrated in the Hijamah areas and also there is less blood in the superficial or outer parts of the body. If Hijamah is done in this condition it can lead to illness and this is also mentioned in some other Ahadeeth which say that Hijamah on a full stomach is disease and on an empty stomach is cure.

When Hijamah is done on a person who has just eaten it often results in vertigo or syncope (fainting).

The second condition is that the **person should have enough strength for the procedure.** This is also proven for the hadith:

The Nabi, upon whom be peace, was cupped while he was fasting. However, if doing this weakens the fasting person, it is disliked. Thabit al-Bunani asked Anas: "Did you dislike

cupping for a fasting person during the time of the Nabi?" He answered: "No [we did not], unless it made someone weak." This is related by al-Bukhari and others.

There are some general conditions which are also recommended:

- The patient should ideally have taken a bath before the procedure, this assists in bringing the blood to the surface and helps it to flow better during the procedure.
- The are where Hijamah is to be done should be shaved, (often this will be done by the Hajjaam)
- The patient should give some sadaqah (charity) beforehand. It is recommended in the Ahadeeth to treat the sick with charity, it prevents calamities and in the case of the Hijamah procedure helps with the procedure being easy and successful.

When should Hijamah be performed?

Hijamah can be performed either in general cases (Hijamah in strength) when the patient is healthy or to treat a particular illness (Hijamah in illness). The times stipulated for these are different.

Hijamah in strength

For general health in those who are suited to cupping, it should be done once a year. During the Spring or Summer time when it is hot is the best season in which to perform Hijamah. The reasons have been described in previous chapters.

Hijamah and the lunar cycle:

In health it is generally recommended to perform Hijamah only on the 17th, 19th or 21st of the lunar month. These are the dates recommended in the Ahadeeth but there is no harm in doing it any time in the latter part of the lunar month from the 17th to the 27th, provided that the climate is suitable for it as detailed above.

The reason for this has to do with the effect of the moon on the blood. Just as the moon has an effect on the sea and produces high tides, in the same manner when the moon is full it brings forth impurities from the blood to the surface of the body and has other effects as well.

it is interesting to note that the term "lunatic" is derived from lunar and indicates the effect of the moon and such behaviour. In fact, lunacy is more likely at the time of the full moon since this is when there is a lot of liver energy which can give rise to easy anger, flared tempers etc.

Many who suffer from conditions such as epilepsy, migraine headaches, high blood pressure etc note that their symptoms are worse during a full moon that at other times of the month. Studies show that more assaults occur around the full moon. More crimes, self and unintentional poisonings and animal bites occur during the full moon cycle as well. The moon also has an impact on fertility, menstruation, and birth rate. Melatonin levels which are influenced by the phase of the moon correlate with the menstrual cycle. Admittance to hospitals and emergency units because of various causes also correlate with the moon phases. In addition, other events associated with human behavior, such as traffic accidents, crimes, and suicides, are more common during the full moon phase as well.

Studies indicate that melatonin and endogenous steroid levels are affected by the phase of the moon and may be the means by which the physiological changes occur in response to the moon phase. The release of these neurohormones may be triggered by the electromagnetic radiation and/or the gravitational pull of the moon.

In a more recent study conducted in 2013 at the Psychiatric Hospital of the University of Basel, Switzerland, researchers found that around the time of full moon, sleep was affected with subjects experiencing decreased electroencephalogram (EEG) activity, taking longer to fall off to sleep, and also reporting decreased sleep quality. This also correlated with lower melatonin levels.

It is however not recommended to have Hijamah during the full moon phase itself, as it is understood that the blood will flow in excessive and unnecessary amounts, but afterwards (from the 17th onward) it is a means of removing the impurities and 'heat' from the body.

Time of day:

It is recommended to perform general Hijamah in the early morning before 10 a.m. while the impurities in the blood are still settled in the areas bled for Hijamah and have not had time to circulate and diffuse in the general circulation. Once the patient starts to get involved in his/her daily activities there is a significant redistribution of blood which is allocated to areas of the body that are in greater need depending on the activity being performed. The patient also may eat something which will cause blood to move to the internal digestive organs.

By the afternoon, the blood starts to recede internally and this is why "blood deficiency" headaches tend to occur at this time. Office workers are especially prone to this and should not be treated with Hijamah after returning from work as this aggravates their blood deficiency issue.

If the patient has had an afternoon nap and is fresh in the evening then Hijamah may be performed provided the climate is hot and the patient has not eaten.

Hijamah in illness

Hijamah in illness can be performed at any time of the month, but it is preferred during the daytime and when the climate is warm or hot.
If this is not possible care should be taken that the room where Hijamah is being performed is warm and there is no draught entering, (whether it be through an incompletely sealed door or window etc.).

The patient should also take extra precaution not to expose themselves to cold after the procedure and neither should they drink or eat cold or raw foods as these will divert heat to the interior of the body. For Hijamah during illness the amount of blood removed must correspond with the level of the pulse and the Hajjaam must have special training in order to apply the procedure effectively to treat the presenting illness. It is better that the treatment is also combined with herbal medication and dietary therapy in such cases.

Body areas for Hijamah

For Hijamah in strength there are 3 main areas as mentioned above for the procedure. These are the head, the area between the shoulder blades and the on the anterior aspect of the foot.

Each of these is relevant to a different constitution though this is a guideline and not a rule.

The head area is more suited to the fire type constitution, the area between the shoulder blades to the wood type and the anterior aspect of the foot to the earth type who suffers from heat in the stomach.

These areas are also proven from the Ahadeeth:

*Anas bin Maalik RadiyAllaahu 'Anhu said: "Rasulullaah SallAllaahu 'Alayhi Wasallam used the treatment of Hijamah on **both sides of his mubaarak neck and between both shoulders, and generally took this treatment** on the seventeenth, nineteenth or the twenty first of the (lunar) month".(Tirmidhi 49:005)*

For Hijamah during illness, the points are not specific and will depend on the condition. The Nabi ﷺ also had this type of Hijamah done as borne out by the following Hadith:

Anas bin Maalik RadiyAllaahu 'Anhu reports: "Sayyidina Rasulullaah SallAllaahu 'Alayhi Wasallam **took treatment of Hijamah on the back of his leg** *at Milal (a place about seventeen miles-27 km-from Madinah Munawwarah in the direction of Makkah) while he was in the state of Ihraam". (Tirmidhi 49:006)*

(Further detail on the points used and the methods for Hijamah during illness is described in the Hijamah treatment guide)

Areas/points that should not be bled

There are a number of areas that should not be bled for the purpose of Hijamah. Some of these lie in close proximity to arteries; others are empirically not suited to bleeding therapies. These include the following areas:

Over the radial artery at the wrist

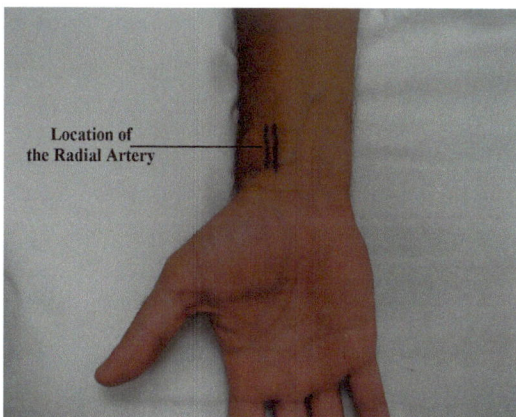

Over the axillary artery (in the armpit)

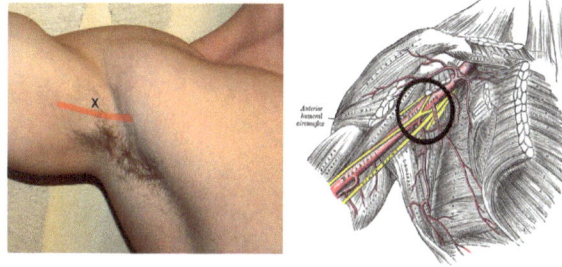

Over the posterior tibial artery

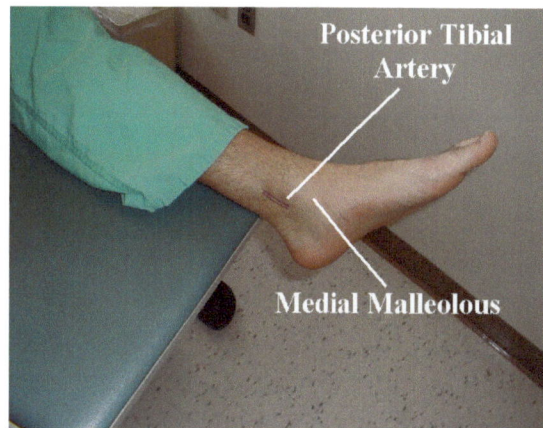

(In Traditional Chinese Medicine this area is connected to the kidney and bleeding here can be detrimental to kidney health)

Over the external iliac artery on the lower abdomen

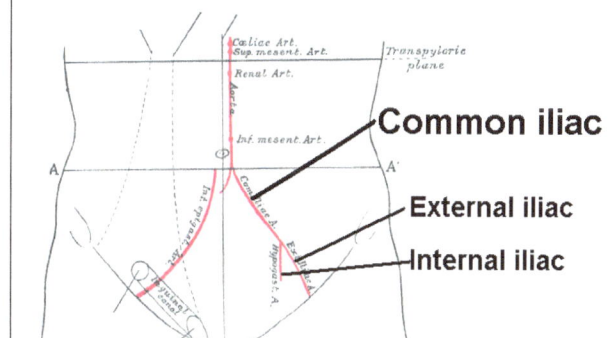

Over the carotid artery in the neck

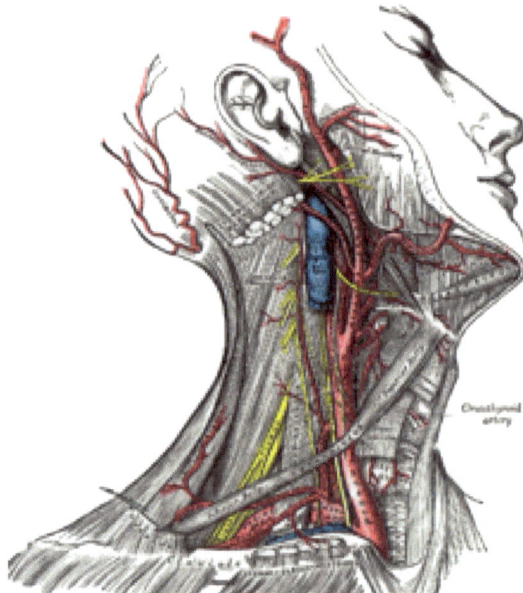

Some areas that overly arteries can be bled but caution must be taken when bleeding so as not to puncture the artery and cause excessive bleeding, these include the dorsalis pedis on the upper aspect of the foot, the superficial temporal artery located at the temples on the head.

How much blood should be removed?

In general Hijamah between 2 to 6 "cups" of blood are removed and this will depend on the constitution of the patient, their current state of health and the change in the color of the blood during the Hijamah procedure.

The constitution is determined as described earlier, with the fire type having the most amount of blood, followed by the liver and earth types.

Feeling the pulse is the best way to determine the current state of health. In general there are three levels of strength to the pulse, these can be described as forceless, normal force and forceful.

In terms of the color of blood, the range is from dark purplish to bright red.

Using these parameters one can determine the amount of blood to be removed in each case by following the table on the next page:

Constitution	Pulse strength	Cups
Earth	Normal	2
Earth	Forceless	0
Earth	Forceful	4
Wood	Normal	4
Wood	Forceless	2
Wood	Forceful	6
Fire	Normal	6
Fire	Forceless	4
Fire	Forceful	8

The third parameter is not used in the table as it overrides the other parameters, which means that If during the Hijamah procedure the blood changes from purple or dark red to a fresh or bright red, the procedure should be stopped and no further blood removed.

What to do after Hijamah?

There are a number of precautions that must be adhered to after the Hijamah procedure. These are essential to prevent infection and also to avoid adverse effects that may occur after the treatment.

The incisions should be cleaned and disinfected appropriately and thereafter covered with a suitable dressing or plaster. I also recommend the use of low-level laser therapy over the incisions to reduce the likelihood of scarring and speed up healing.

The body is in a condition of vulnerability after Hijamah and care must be taken to avoid exposure to cold as well as the weakness that arises from not eating appropriately after Hijamah. For this reason it is recommended to cover the body appropriately after Hijamah especially if the weather may be cold or damp. There is also the possibility of blood clots developing if the patient remains immobile afterward, one should therefore not go to sleep immediately afterwards but rather take a short walk and remain active for a few hours before resting.

Recommended foods include those that are rich in healthy fats and proteins and these should be taken one hour after the Hijamah. Plenty of fluids should be taken to redress the loss of body fluids, but refrain from caffeine and sugary drinks.

Hijamah patients should also avoid showering immediately after the procedure and take care not to scratch the incisions as this will contribute to scarring. The dressing should be changed daily or as needed until the wound has completely healed.

The practitioner should dispose of the instruments used and the blood in an appropriate manner to avoid cross infection. Many cases of Hepatitis and HIV have been reported as a result of mishandling of medical waste. The ideal situation is that the cups used are buried irrespective of whether they are glass or plastic cups. It is possible to sterilise glass cups but the preference would still be to bury them or dispose of them in special medical waste disposal facilities. Prospective patients can also take their own cups to the Hajjaam to ensure that Hijamah is not being administered to them using cups that were used on other patients before them.

There are a number of different techniques that can be employed when performing Hijama or bloodletting. These include bleeding with or without using suction and the bleeding of superficial skin areas or veins or the bleeding of points on the ear or extremities. These methods will be described in this section after the basic precautions and safety procedures are detailed.

Sterile equipment

The most important aspect of practicing bloodletting is to use sterile equipment. Do not use reuse the same equipment if it is not absolutely sterile. As mentioned in previous chapters there are numerous cases of infection that have occurred due to Hijama being practiced with unsterilised equipment. The best practice is to use disposable single use cups and bleeding equipment for the procedure.

Some therapists ask patients to bring their own cups and then give them back to the patient after the procedure. This also should not be done as you do not have any control over those cups.

Infection will spread from those cups to other members of the family and friends that come into contact with that equipment.

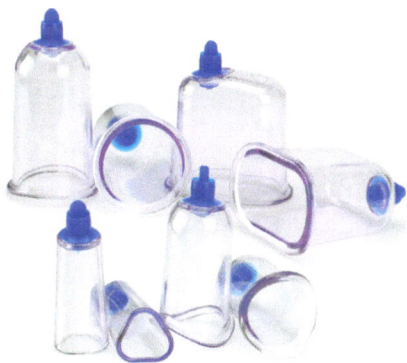

With regards to the plastic suction cups that are widely used today, please understand that if these are used for collecting blood during a bloodletting procedure then they must be discarded as they cannot be sterilised due to the valve mechanism in the cup.

If you are using glass cups and reusing surgical blade equipment then it is possible to sterilise these with an autoclave, or using medical solutions specifically produced for sterilisation. If these are not available you can do one of the following:

1. Place them in gently boiling water for 30 minutes, (but this may not eliminate some bacterial "spores" and could cause issues with rusting over time, especially on sharp instruments like scissors or knives.) Note: always sterilize scissors and clamps in the "open" position.

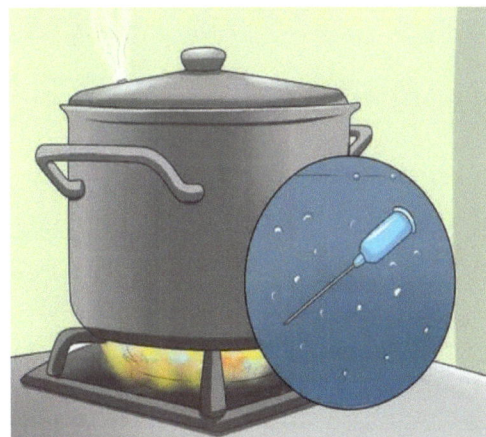

2. Soaking in bleach (Sodium or Calcium Hypochlorite). 15-30 minutes in a 0.1% solution of bleach will disinfect instruments but no longer or rusting will occur. Instruments must be rinsed in sterilized water afterward.

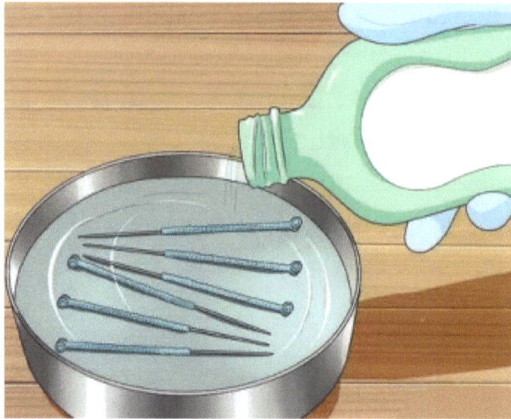

3. Soaking in 70% isopropyl alcohol for 30 minutes is another option.

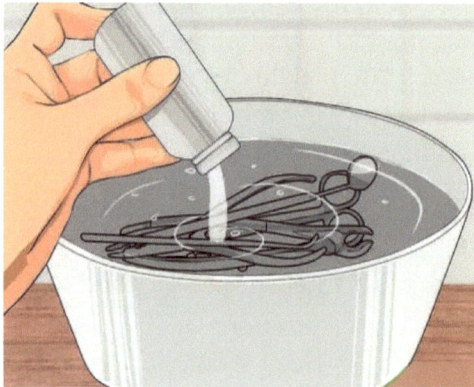

4. A good method that I suggest is to put instruments in a metal tray with alcohol and ignite them. The flame and alcohol, or even just fire itself (if evenly distributed) will do the job, but eventually causes damage to the instruments. When performing this method of sterilisation please ensure that you do not use too much alcohol as this will create a larger flame. Fire makes things pure and it is the best method, the cups and other instruments should first be washed and brushed clean.

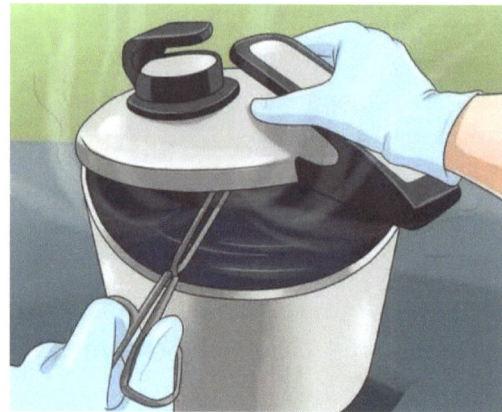

Please note that this refers to the flammable chemical alcohol, not the alcohol that is erroneously understood as liquor or wine which will be impure and not permissible to use for this purpose.

Disposal of medical waste

Blood and other medical waste should be disposed of appropriately using the appropriate sharps and medical waste bins and companies that deal specifically with this type of waste. If this is not possible at all then the blood and contaminated biowaste should be buried appropriately. This is not only a hygiene and safety concern but Islamically it is correct that blood should be buried as is the case with all other parts of the body such as the hair and nails etc.

For this purpose a large biowaste container should be kept close to where the treatment is being performed so that the waste products can be placed immediately into these bins during the procedure. Normally these are coloured yellow but it may differ in your country.

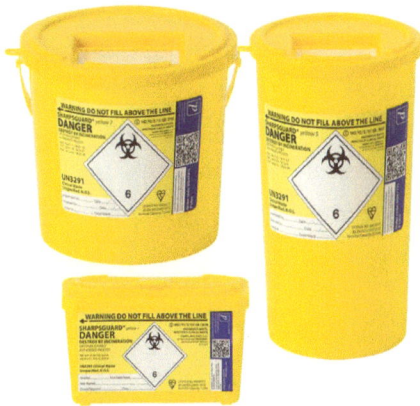

Using gloves

The primary purpose of surgical gloves is to act as a protective barrier to prevent possible transmission of diseases between healthcare professionals and patients during surgical and bloodletting procedures.

There are two types of gloves available on the market and you should be certain that you use the correct type. Medical examination gloves are generally not intended for surgical procedures whereas surgical gloves are to be used when performing Hijama as it is a surgical procedure.

Note on Materials

Natural rubber latex surgical gloves were first used in 1890. Their usage increased dramatically in the late 1980s, when latex gloves were widely recommended to prevent transmission of blood- borne infections, such as the human immunodeficiency virus (HIV).

The incidence of allergic reactions to latex began to rise rapidly among patients and health care workers in the 1990s. Since then, new synthetic glove materials have been introduced, which have differing properties with regards to strength, comfort and sensitivity. However, the majority of surgical gloves are still made from latex.

Synthetic materials are also available though some do not provide adequate protection against chemicals and blood products.

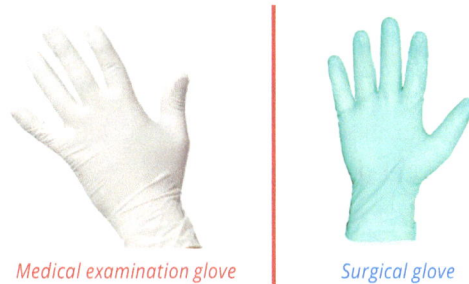

Medical examination glove   *Surgical glove*

Fainting

During Hijama treatment, the patient may feel faint. The procedure and the sensations it may cause should therefore be carefully explained before starting.

For those about to receive Hijama for the first time, treatment in a lying position is preferred. The complexion should be closely watched and the pulse frequently checked to detect any untoward reactions as early as possible.

Symptoms of impending faintness include feeling unwell, a sensation of giddiness, movement or swaying of surrounding objects, and weakness. An oppressive feeling in the chest, palpitations, nausea and sometimes vomiting may ensue. The complexion usually turns pale and the pulse is weak. In severe cases, there may be coldness of the extremities, cold sweats, a fall in blood pressure, and loss of consciousness. Such reactions are often due to nervousness, hunger, fatigue, extreme weakness of the patient, an unsuitable position, or too forceful manipulation.

If warning symptoms appear, make the patient lie flat if they are not already doing so, if this does not provide relief, remove any cups immediately and let the patient lie with the head down and the legs raised, as the symptoms are probably due to a transient, insufficient blood supply to the brain. Offer warm sweet drinks.

The symptoms usually disappear after a short rest.

In severe cases, first aid should be given and, when the patient is medically stable, you can press the revive consciousness point. The patient will usually respond rapidly to these measures, but if the symptoms persist, emergency medical assistance will be necessary.

Hijama Equipment

The following is the equipment that you will need in order to perform the Hijama procedures that are taught in this course:

Bleeding equipment:

Lancing devices

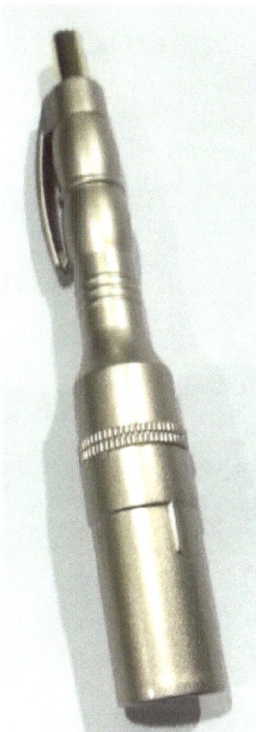

A lot of therapists use a surgical or general blade (non-sterile) but I prefer to use a lancing device as it does not leave scars and also the flow of blood is controlled. In the past only actual blades were used so this is also acceptable but practicing in the modern climate means taking into account the considerations of scars, keloid etc which is elimiated when using a lancet. The lancet device uses multiple lancets to make opening in the skin which are sufficient for blood to escape.

By using this device over multiple points with 5 incisions being made each time for a total of about 30 incisions and then allowing the blood to flow as per the individuals own blood pressure and need to express the blood, this facilitates the best and most effective Hijama release.

Individual lancets

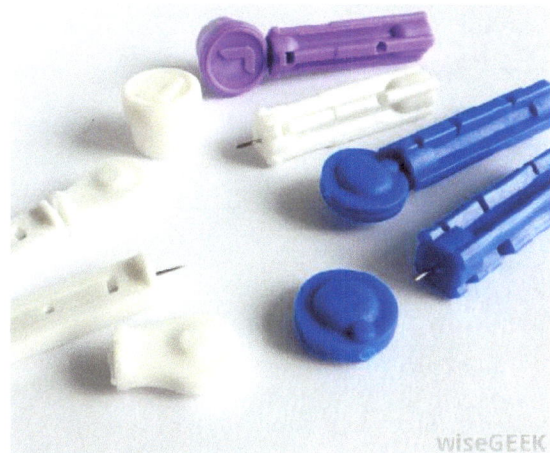

Lacets are required for the lancing device and they are often easy to use for opening spider veins without piercing the other side of the vein and causing internal bleeding.

Surgical blades

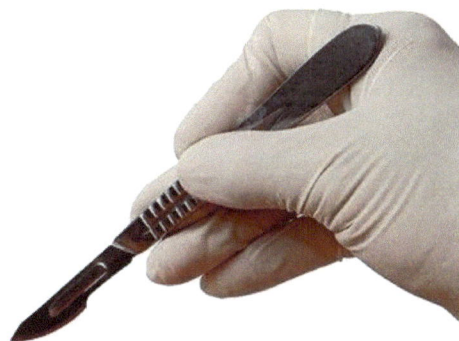

Surgical blades are useful when one cannot use a lancing device and also for practicing the other advanced methods of bleeding spider veins etc. Using this blade however is more dangerous as one can easily damage internal structures and also cause more bleeding than is desired.

Plum blossom needle

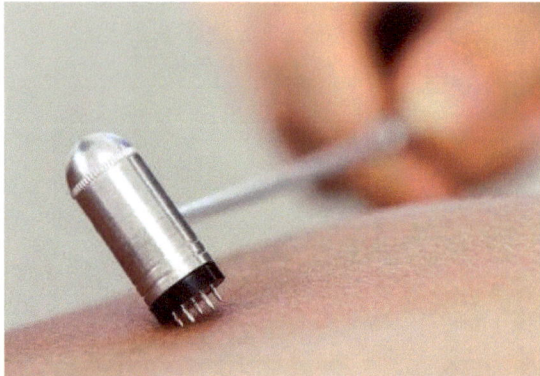

This is a tool used a lot in Chinese Medical therapies that has 7 piercing points on it and is used to accomplish the effect of drawing blood to an area and then releasing it through Hijama.

Other equipment

Bleeding equipment is specific to Hijama while the remaining equipment and supplies are used generally in medical practices and should be common to you by now, these include:

• Surgical gloves

• Sharps bins - 1 for blood and a seperate smaller 1 for sharps at least

• Treatment bed or chair for the patient to rest on during and after the procedure

• Bed sheets

• Bed lining - to prevent the sheets from getting stained with blood

• Paper towels - these are useful when removing the cups to avoid patients blood from soiling the bed

• Surgical trays for used blades etc

• Cotton wool buds

• Surgical plasters for covering the incisions

• Plastic or glass cups

• Pump for plastic cups

• Hair trimmer/shaver for removing hair when necessary

• Forceps for fire cupping

• Mini-blow torch or lighter

• Towels

Preparing the patient for Hijama

Once you have determined that no contraindications are present for performing Hijama on the patient you now need to prepare the patient for the procedure. By now you should have made sure that the patient had not had anything to eat for at least the last 2 hours, especially if you are doing general/sunnah Hijama.

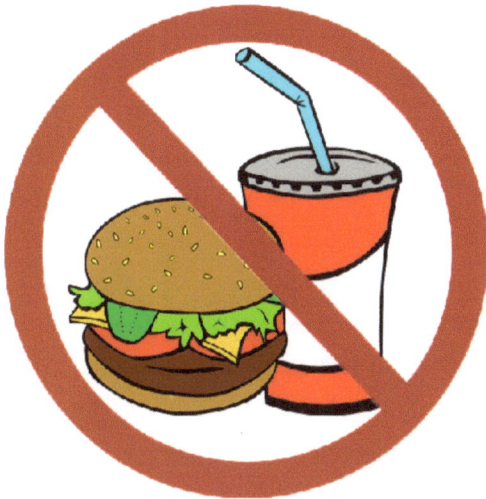

You may still do other methods of Hijama that do not involve drawing a lot of blood, i.e point bleeding if the patient has eaten soon before the treatment.

The room in which Hijama is being done should be warm. There should be no cold draft entering the room as this is detrimental and will cause an invasion of wind and cold into the body which is weakened during and after the Hijama process. This is a common

cause of infection in hospitals and doctors rooms and most practitioners are very neglectful of exposure to cold wind whether it be natural or from an airconditioner. You

should also be careful that when the patient leaves the room they are not exposed to cold wind as well, They should be appropriately dressed when leaving and counselled to stay away from cold wind especially.

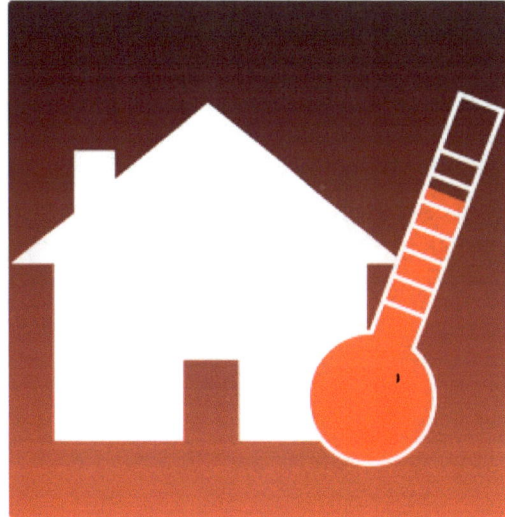

Depending on which area or point you are going to perform the procedure you need to advise and assist the patient to remove that much of the clothing which is necessary to perform the procedure. They should also be either seated or laying down in such a way that gives you easy access to the location needed.

Once they are laying in the correct position, you should use a disinfectant on the area to be bled and then continue with the

procedure that you are performing which will be explained in the next sections.

Bleeding techniques

When bleeding a **point** or a **larger** area you have a few considerations viz.

• How much blood to remove

This will be guided by your diagnosis and also the general use of the point/area itself and it may be from a few drops to a large sized cup or more than one cup. When bleeding a point it is often as a combination of many points selected to address the problem so one does not always need to remove a lot of blood from each point. Whereas when you are bleeding an area you may want to remove more blood especially if the patient has a strong constitution and you are doing a general Hijama treatment.

The best guide with regard to the quantity of blood that should be removed are

1. The natural flow of blood (i.e allowing the cup to fill until the clotting of the blood itself stops the bleeding)
2. The amplitude of the pulse wave in the nearest palpable artery (if you have been trained in pulse diagnosis)

• Whether to use a vacuum cup to draw blood, allow it to flow freely or encourage it with the use of manual techniques

This is related to the previous discussion. The point between the eyebrows for example as well as other such points that have similar anatomy can be pinched and squeezed after bleeding to encourage flow of more drops of blood. A small cup may also be used but will leave a mark on the patients face for some time and this should be taken into consideration. Sometimes a cup may not adhere to the skin adequately so this also has to be considered.

Many self-taught Hijama therapists insist on the use of fire cupping claiming it to be the only way as it is the traditional way, but actually in the period of the Prophet ﷺ it was common practice to use horns of animals as the "cupping" device whereas fire cupping is a later invention. Nevertheless there is benefit in the fire cupping method in that the heat assists in drawing out blood allowing it to flow more easily. I generally prefer the use of plastic disposable cups however as it reduces the likelihood of an accident occurring in practice and the suction can be adjusted during the treatment, this not being possible with glass fire cups.

• What bleeding instrument to use

My preference is to use a lancet or multiple lancet device for point and also area bleeding but there are cases where the blade may be better,

specifically for area bleeding when one wants to target veins directly or the patient has poor blood flow and one wants to encourage more bleeding. The underlying structures must be considered when performing Hijama on points located on the head and temples, the arms, the feet, the face and the hands. When using a lancet there are also multiple techniques that can be applied.

Technique guide:

1. First locate the point/area to be bled

2. Sterilise the area

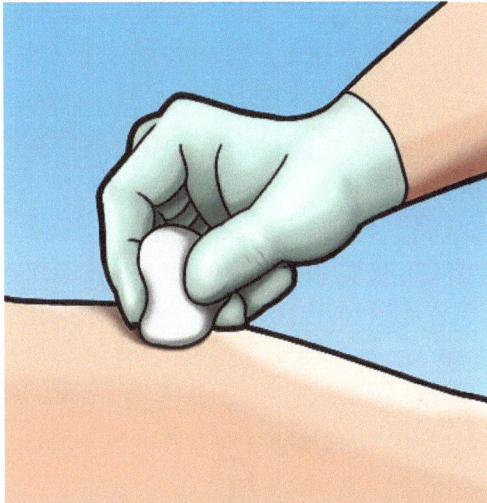

3. If you will be using a cup you can apply the cup with some suction in order to bring blood to the point/area. (this is before making incisions in the skin)

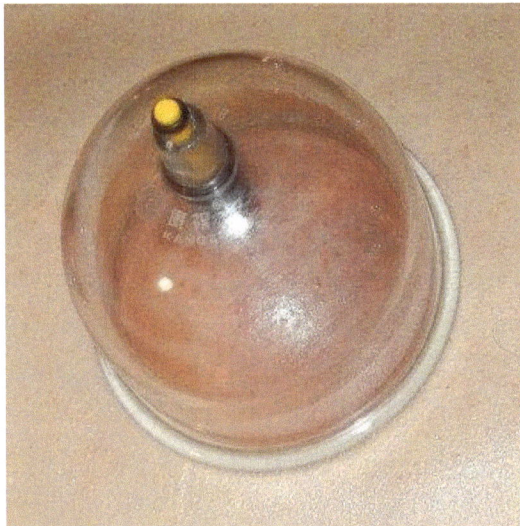

4. Once the point/area has drawn sufficient blood, indicated by a change in the skin color to a light red or sometimes purplish, remove the cup.

5. Without too much delay, bleed the point/area using either an individual lancet or multi lancet device or a surgical blade

   1. If using a single lancet it may be useful to pinch the skin up and then insert the tip of the lancet. The lancet tip should not be "dragged" or "scarped" on the skin as if one is cutting with the lancet. The lancet is not meant to be a blade that one uses to cut, if this is done it causes unnecessary pain. It is meant for a quick and straight insertion and removal.

   2. If using a multi lancet device be careful not to apply too deeply on areas with thin skin and underlying structures which are close to the surface, such as the scalp region, some areas of the face, the wrist region, the ankles, the knees and elbows, the ear and the neck region (where I do not recommend the multi lancet be used at all),

   3. If you choose to use a surgical blade, carefully make multiple short incisions in the circular mark left by the suction of the cup keeping these to the inner two thirds of the mark. Do not make long incisions, each should be no more than 4mm in length.

6. Allow the blood to flow freely, or massage and pinch the surrounding skin to encourage more flow or otherwise re-apply acup to remove a more significant amount of blood

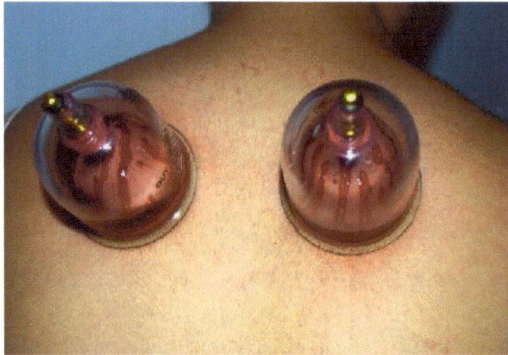

7. When you are satisfied, remove the cup if placed, clean off the excess blood. Then you can reswab the area to sterilise and apply a bandage if necessary or leave if there is no bleeding.

8. Apply some moxa or laser heat to the point for 5 to 20 seconds (especially for patients exhibiting signs of weakness)

9. Continue to the next point/area to be used or do the next point while the previous is drawing blood.

During the procedure you should always check with the patient how they are feeling in order to establish if they are conscious and if they are managing the treatment. Some patients may feel unwell during the treatment and may even faint, you need to be prepared for this. If the patient is lying down you may not notice and for this reason you should be communicating with the patient. It is not absolutely necessary to remove the cups if the patient faints but if it progresses to pallor, perspiration etc then the cups should be calmly removed, bandage applies and the patient treated for shock.

Some points that you may want to bleed are located on the extremities and these should be bled carefully taking into account the sensitivity and also the proximity of underlying structures.

There are two types of points on the extremities and they have different considerations, those located at the tips or around the nails of the fingers and toes and those located more distally (closer to the body).

The points located on the tips of the fingers and toes and close to or at the corners of the nailbed should only be bled with a single lancet or very carefully with the tip of a surgical blade. Only a few drops of blood should be removed by pinching the skin around.

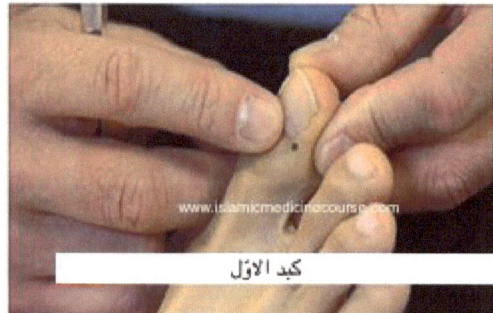

كبد الاوّل

These types of points (at the toes or fingers) tend to have a drastic action of reducing heat and energy/qudra from the top part of the body and are therefore effective in emergency situations that are characterised by heat and excess, examples include epileptic fits where the patient has a red face and there is a lot of movement or cases where there is a severe headache together with red eyes, red face, extreme thirst and irritability.

When piercing this point 3 to 7 drops of blood can be removed. Using a lancet here is tricky as the skin is very thin and the underlying structures close to the surface. Be careful when piercing the skin, pierce at an angle, not directly vertically and do not go too deep, only a small prick will be required to cause some blood to be released, more bleeding can be encouraged by rubbing around the point and squeezing the point or the whole finger or toe.

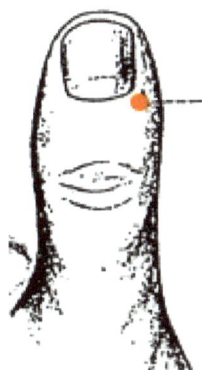

Bleeding veins and varicosities

Some of the points in this atlas indicate identifying a small vein that may be present in the area and bleeding this vein. This is an advanced technique in Hijama that practitioners should be aware of.

Low back pain vein

This vein will appear behind the knee in the popliteal fossa when a person suffers from poor circulation causing low back pain and maybe even other gynecological and menstrual problems.

There are two approaches here, one is to look for the vein in response to a complaint of the lower back region and the other is to look for the vein as part of a general examination. In both cases if it is found there will be benefit in bleeding it even if the patient does not have any related symptoms.

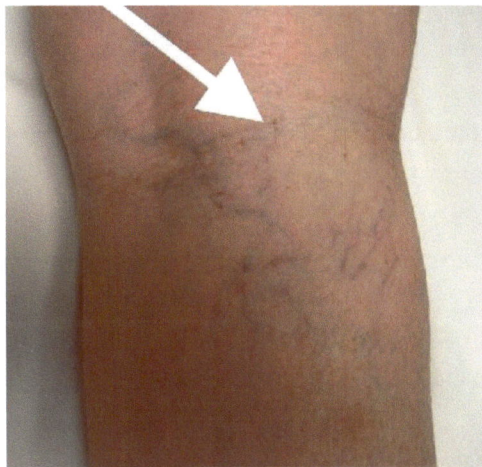

In the picture above you can see that there are many subcutaneous veins that are visible. Some are thicker than others, the general rule is that we do not pierce the very thick veins which are the typical varicose veins. We prefer to bleed thinner veins that are more red than purple. In the picture here the arrow points to the vein that is the prime candidate for bleeding. It is located midway in the popliteal crease.

The method of bleeding is to pierce it with a lancet but only sufficiently to open the top part of the vein. The lancet should not go all the way through and pierce the bottom of the vein as this will cause bleeding into the tissues which is not desired. We want the blood to be released to the surface of the body.

3 to 7 drops can be removed in this way and often the effects are miraculous for those who are suffering from acute lower back pain.

Spider veins

Similar looking veins called spider veins or spider naevi can often be found in other areas where the patient may be experiencing chronic pain. In fact the appearance of these spider naevi only occurs after chronic blood stasis. They can be seen in the shoulder region of bodybuilders with chronic shoulder pain and weakness, they can also be found on the lower back region and at other places as well.

If you find these in an area of a pain complaint by a patient then they are worth treating. Choose 3 to 5 such fine, reddish or reddish purple veins and "nick" them lightly with a lancet to remove blood. DO NOT place a cup over to extract blood as the cup edges will block the veins and you will not get venous blood that you need to remove in these cases. For each vein 3 to 7 drops of blood should be removed.

When you have completed the bleeding of a particular point/area you will be left with incisions that may or may not still be bleeding. These have to be appropriately cared for both immediately after the treatment and afterward as well. If not done they may become infected, lead to scarring or keloids or cause other complications.

Lancet cuts

When using lancets most often the incisions are not prone to continuous bleeding after the procedure.

In either case the first step is to sterilise the area. Thereafter heat in the form of an infrared heat lamp or moxa can be applied especially in patients with a weaker constitution (the detailed use of moxa and heating therapies is discussed in other short courses of mine).

You do not need to apply a dressing or medical plaster over lancet cuts unless the cuts are still bleeding. They heal very quickly (within 2 to 5 days) and do not commonly present a problem afterwards. They also are unlikely to leave scars or develop keloid.

An exception to this is where one has used multiple lancets to do Hijama on the back or other large areas, in this case it is still prudent to use at least a medical plaster over the area bled. The round type plasters can be used or any other type that covers all the lancet "cuts".

The patient can take a bath soon after the procedure in the case of using lancets where the bleeding has already stopped. However in the case of a surgical blade where the cuts may still be bleeding or have the possibility of doing so, the bath should be delayed.

3 edged needle/surgical blade

The 3 edge needle and surgical blade leaves a larger wound in the skin that will generally require a dressing/plaster to be applied. These incisions can take up to 2 weeks to heal fully.

A honey wound dressing is recommended and available from www.aconitemedical.com

The patient may notice some soreness, tenderness, tingling, numbness, and itching around the incision. There may also be mild oozing and bruising, and a small lump may form. This is normal and no cause for concern.

However the patient should be advised to seek medical care if any of the following occurs:

- A yellow or green discharge
- An increase in the size of the incision.
- Redness or hardening of the surrounding area.
- The incision is hot to the touch.
- Fever.
- Increasing or unusual pain.
- Excessive bleeding that has soaked through the dressing/plaster

Scars can be prevented from occurring if the practitioner administers low level laser therapy a few days to a week after the procedure. LLLT reduces the likelihood of scar and keloid formation.

The patient is advised not to bath immediately and delay for at least 6 after using this method of bleeding as the heat encourages increased bleeding and delayed healing time. It will be better if a period of 24 hours is kept before doing so.

Hijama Points Guide

In the following section I have prepared a guide to the most effective points to be used for Hijama. Together with this I have also written what the point is good for, how to use it and what precautions there are when doing so.

The videos recordings of each point are available to you by going to my website and registering your purchase of this manual, go to www.drlatib.com and click books, then register manual purchase to get access to the video series.

Brain function points

Location: 4 points, 2 of these located 1 finger breadth lateral on the line between the two ear apex points. and the other 2 being directly in front of and behind the head summit point along the midline.

Functions: Stimulates brain activity, increases blood flow to the CNS.

Indications: Poor memory, alzheimers, dementia, Parkinson's, insomnia

Method: Each point can be pierced and allowed to bleed freely or a small cup can be used to draw a minimal amount of blood.

Comments: These points and method are preferred in patients who are deficient in blood (as opposed to using Head Summit)

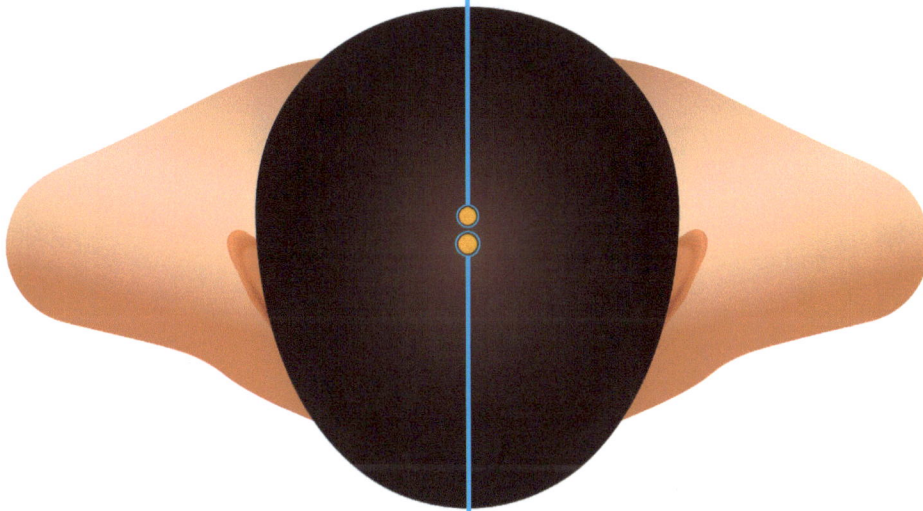

Head summit - قمة الرأس

Location: At the vertex of the head. Can be found by folding the ears and running a line from the tip of one ear to the other, the point will be where it intersects the midline. (A slight depression can often be felt here)

Functions: Removes heat from the head, clears fire from the liver.

Indications: Headache, dizziness, eye pain and redness, irritability, hypertension from excess heat in the upper body. All pain conditions in the head due to heat or blood stasis

Method: Multiple incisions with a lancet or blade followed by using a medium to large cup in those with a strong constitution. Point bleeding can also be done in combination with the four flowers points for those with a deficiency (blood) constitution or syndrome. (Do not use a cup on this point for patients with severe blood deficiency)

Ear apex (anti-inflammatory) point

Location: At the tip of the apex of the ear. Easily located with the posterior half of the ear folded forward, the point is located at the highest point of the superior crease.

Functions: Treats allergic conditions and acute inflammation as well as acute high blood pressure. Reduces excess heat syndromes.

Indications: acute allergy, sore throat due to infection, severe headache, red eyes, high fever.

Method: Pierce the point with a lancet and squeeze 20 to 50 drops of blood out on each ear.

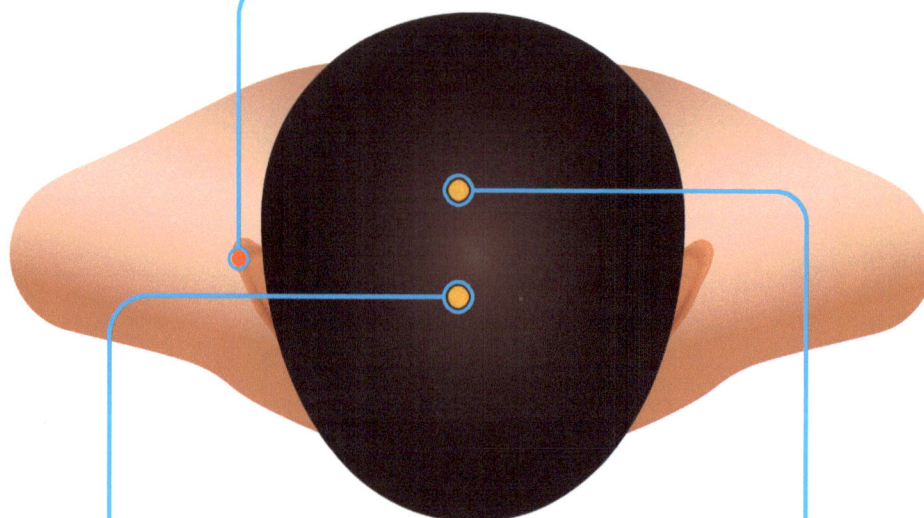

Epilepsy point

Location: Two finger breadths in front of the Head Summit point.

Functions: Treats epilepsy due to heat and phlegm heat affecting the mind.

Method: Multiple incisions with a lancet or blade followed by using a medium to large cup in those with a strong constitution.

Mania point

Location: Two finger breadths behind the Head Summit point

Functions: Treats manic behaviour, restlessness and anxiety due to heat and may be also phlegm affecting the mind.

Method: Multiple incisions with a lancet or blade followed by using a medium to large cup in those with a strong constitution.

Sinus point

Location: One finger breadth in front of the anterior hairline.

Functions: Clears heat from the sinuses and eyes.

Indications: nasal congestion, rhinitis, nasal polyps, sinus headache. Eye/Vision issues - shortsightedness, visual dizziness, painful/red eyes. Facial swelling.

Method: Multiple incisions with a lancet or blade followed by using a medium to large cup in those with a strong constitution.

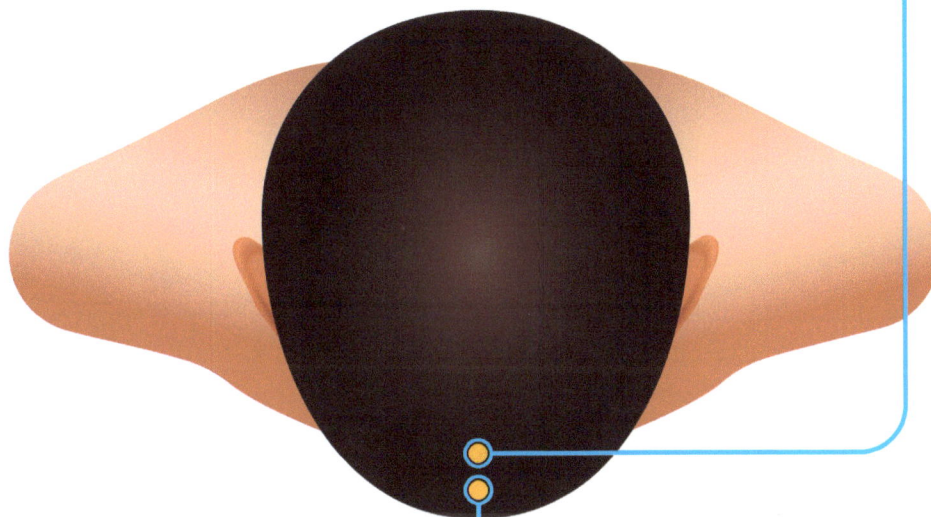

Special Ruqya point 1

Location: half a finger breadth in front of the anterior hairline.

Functions: it has the same functions as the sinus point but is more effective for headache. This point however has a connection with the metaphysical and can be used when there is an element of sihr that is producing headaches or other symptoms such as mania and depression. It is normally sensitive when the sihr or jinn has been present for a long time and has resulted in chronic phlegm affecting the mind.

Method: Multiple incisions with a lancet or blade followed by using a medium to large cup in those with a strong constitution.

Head corner

Location: It is located half a finger within the anterior hairline at the corner of the forehead.

Functions: It is used for splitting headaches; headache with nausea and vomiting; headache with eye pain (migraine) - particularly when these headaches are frontal headaches. Also for poor vision, twitching eyelids, eyepain, excessive tearing and dizziness. In terms of syndromes it addresses wind in the head that is associated with heat in the stomach, therefore can be associated with symptoms of stomach heat such as headache worse for hunger, halitosis, bleeding gums etc.

Method: For pure excess conditions a small cup can be used. For poor vision, twitching eyelids and dizziness due to blood deficiency use a blade or lancet only to release a few drops of blood or otherwise use a Hijama puncture needle if you are trained in it.

Special ruqya point 2

Location: 5 finger breadths within the hairline of the forehead, 3 finger breadths lateral to the midline.

Functions: Regulates the Liver/ GallBladder, Clears Wind, Calms the Mind. Treats Sihr and effects of Jinn.

Indications: Stiff Neck, Headache, Epilepsy. Used on the (R) side for psychological conditions such as anxiety and depression and on the (L) side for attention related conditions such as ADD/ADHD. Also useful for issues which come from sir or jinn influences.

Method: Multiple incisions with a lancet or blade followed by using a small cup.

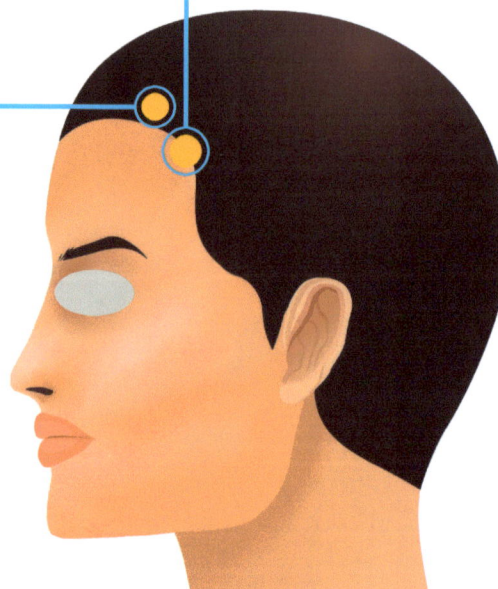

Above the ear Migraine point

Location: In the temporal region, in the slight depression 1 finger breadth directly above the apex of the ear.

Functions: Migraine, one-sided or unilateral headaches and associated nausea, vomiting a/or visual disturbances. Also treats headaches due to alcohol consumption, drug use and medication side effects. Also treats cases of continuous vomiting that is due to a heat in the gallbladder type syndrome.

Method: Multiple incisions with a lancet or blade followed by using a small cup.

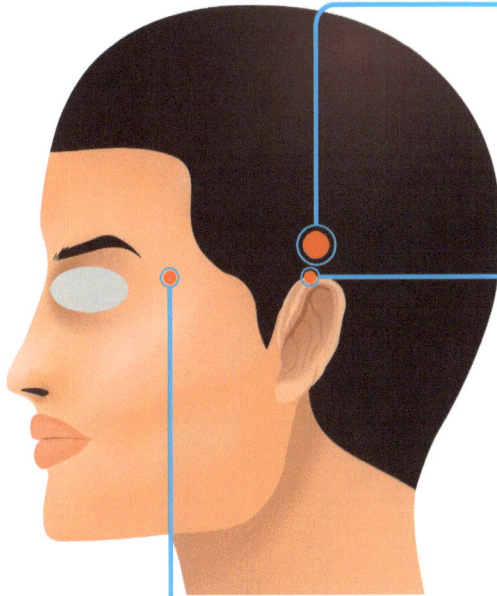

Ear apex (anti-inflammatory) point

Location: At the tip of the apex of the ear. Easily located with the posterior half of the ear folded forward, the point is located at the highest point of the ear when folded

Functions: Treats allergic conditions and acute inflammationas well as acute high blood pressure.Reduces excess heat syndromes.

Indications: acute allergy, sore throat due to infection,severe headache, red eyes, high fever.

Method: Pierce the point with a lancet and squeeze 20 to 50 drops of blood out from each ear.

Temple point

Location: In the depression at the centre of the temple, about 1 finger breadth posterior to the midpoint between the lateral end of the eyebrow and the outer canthus of the eye.

Function: When bled this point reduces pain, inflammation and swelling as well as heat from the liver pathways and organ.

Indications: Temporal, one-sided a/or migraine headaches. Eye issues - pain, swelling, redness, photophobia, visual acuity.Local point for toothache, facial paralysis, pain, etc. Empirical point for swelling of the breasts (Mastitis)

Method: Bleed with a lancet taking care to avoid puncturing blood vessels which are present in this region. In strong constitutions a small cup can be placed here.

Comments: This area often throbs during a headache and is one of the locations for performing pulse diagnosis (see pulsediagnosiscourse.com). If you are not confident of avoiding the blood vessel do not bleed this point.

Head summit - قمة الرأس

Location: At the vertex of the head. Can be found by folding the ears and running a line from the tip of one ear to the other, the point will be where it intersects the midline. (A slight depression can often be felt here)

Functions: Removes heat from the head, clears fire from the liver.

Indications: Headache, dizziness, eye pain and redness, irritability, hypertension from excess heat in the upper body. All pain conditions in the head due to heat or blood stasis

Method: Multiple incisions with a lancet or blade followed by using a medium to large cup in those with a strong constitution. Point bleeding can also be done in combination with the four flowers points for those with a deficiency (blood) constitution or syndrome. (Do not use a cup on this point for patients with severe blood deficiency)

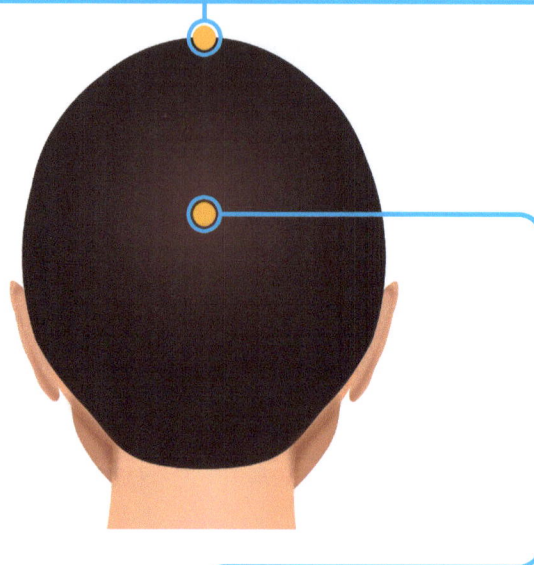

Qamahduwa depression (Sunnah point) - جوزة القمحدوة

Location: In the depression midway between the vertex and the nape hairline.

Discussion: This point has been mentioned in the ahadeeth and commented on by the scholars in the past. The hadeeth mention that Hijama in this point cures 72 types of ailments. However warnings are also sounded in the books of hadeeth regarding the fact that this location is where the memory of a person resides and if Hijama is done without need, without a condition where blood is in excess then this can and has resulted in loss of memory. This is why it is essential to determine if the condition is one of "excess" blood. If a "dryness" of blood condition is present then this point should not be used. (For more details on how to identify excess and deficiency blood syndromes see my courses at www.drlatib.com)

Functions: Treats excess liver diseases and calms anger, temper and jinn or sir related mania or schizophrenia.

Treats: Stiff neck, headache.Visual dizziness, blurring of vision. Epilepsy, Insomnia, Manic Depression.

Method: Multiple incisions with a lancet or blade followed by using a small to medium cup.

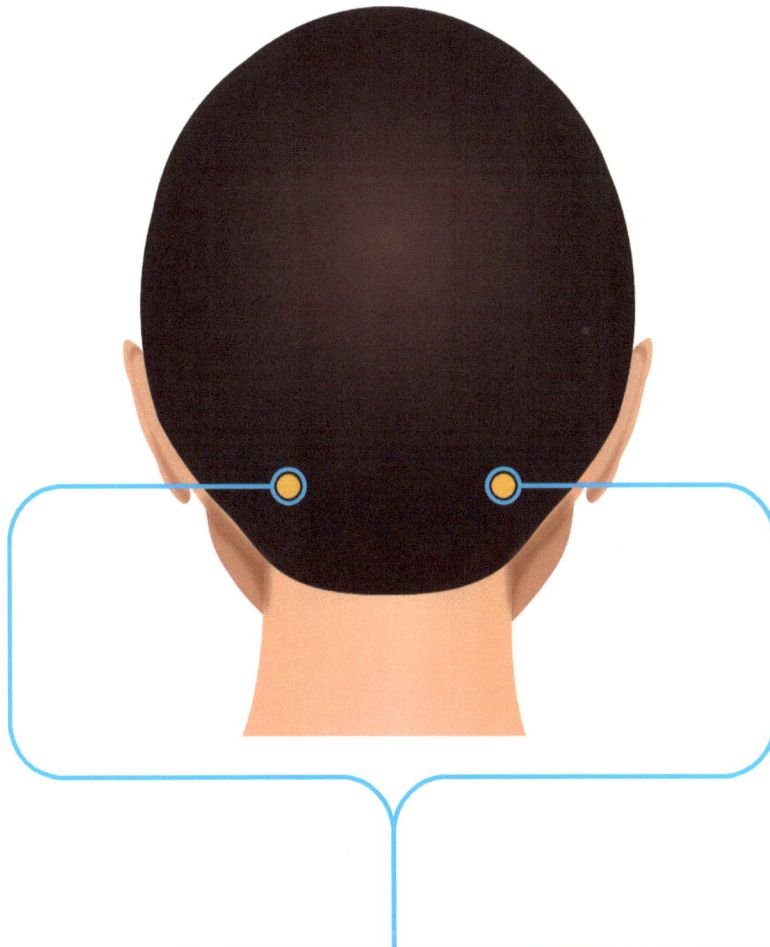

اخدعان

Location: In the depression between the upper portion of the sternocleidomastoid muscle and the trapezius

Functions: Releases acute infections from the upper respiratory tract. Lowers heat and pressure in the head. Relaxes the mind and relieves tension especially due to heat rising in the liver

Treats: fever/chills, stiff neck; paralysis, twitching, tremors, numbness, dizziness, vertigo. seizures, mental/neurological face, throat and sense organs heat, Headache, especially occipital. Treats eye issues. pain, weakness, stiffness of the neck and upper back
Hypertension.

●**Note:** This is a point that is recorded in the ahadeeth as being recommended for Hijama. (Ibn Majah)

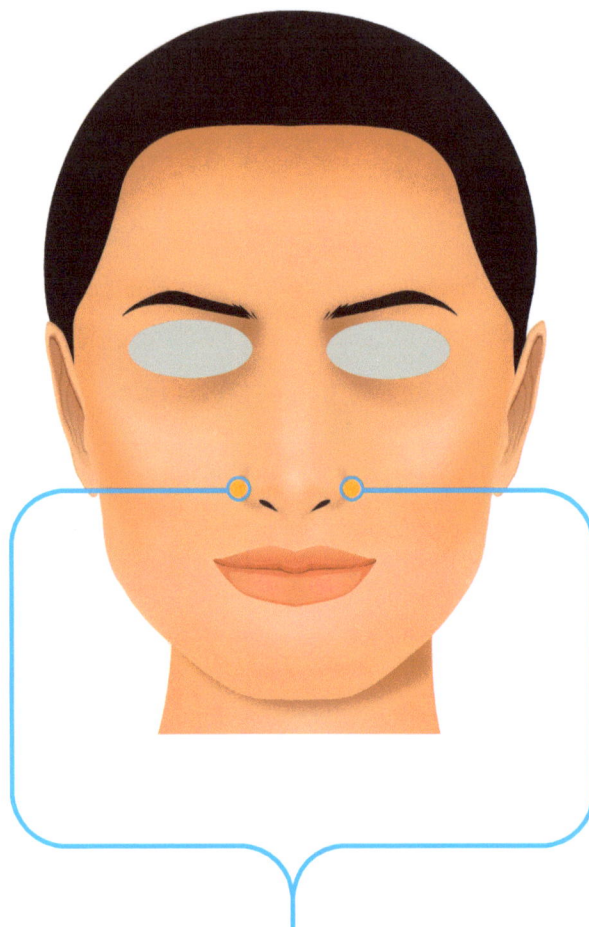

Nasal clearance

Location: In the nasolabial groove, level with the midpoint of the lateral border of the ala nasi.

Functions: Clears heat and congestion from the nasal sinuses.

Indiactions: Treats loss of smell or taste, nasal discharge, any nose a/or sinus issues, nasal polyps, rhinitis, sinusitis, allergies

Method: Use a lancet or very small blade edge to make small incisions and then allow to bleed or use a small cup to remove more blood if the patient has clear heat excess signs. *(Be careful not make deep and long incisions here as they may leave scars, only perform if you are able to do very fine, very small incisions. it will be better to use a lancet only although the cuts should be very shallow, you can pinch the skin up in this area if possible while making the incisions)*

Forehead relief

Location: Directly in line with the pupil of the eye, 1.5 finger breadths above the ridge of the eyebrow

Functions: Clears heat from the forehead and eyes. Relieves pain

Indications: Frontal/temporal headaches
Eye conditions - redness, swelling, itching, twitching, etc.

Method: This point can be bled either with a medium or small cup or a few drops can be removed depending on the nature of the illness. If it is an acute and severe headache with primarily excess heat signs then a medium or small cup can be used on each point. If it is a chronic headache situation with signs of blood deficiency then a small cup must be used in order to provide relief of pain but not aggravate the blood deficiency. For eye diseases the method is similar except that it can be bled more regularly with a few drops of blood removed each time to control recurring eye conditions. Since this point is on the face care must be taken to use an incision method that will not leave scars

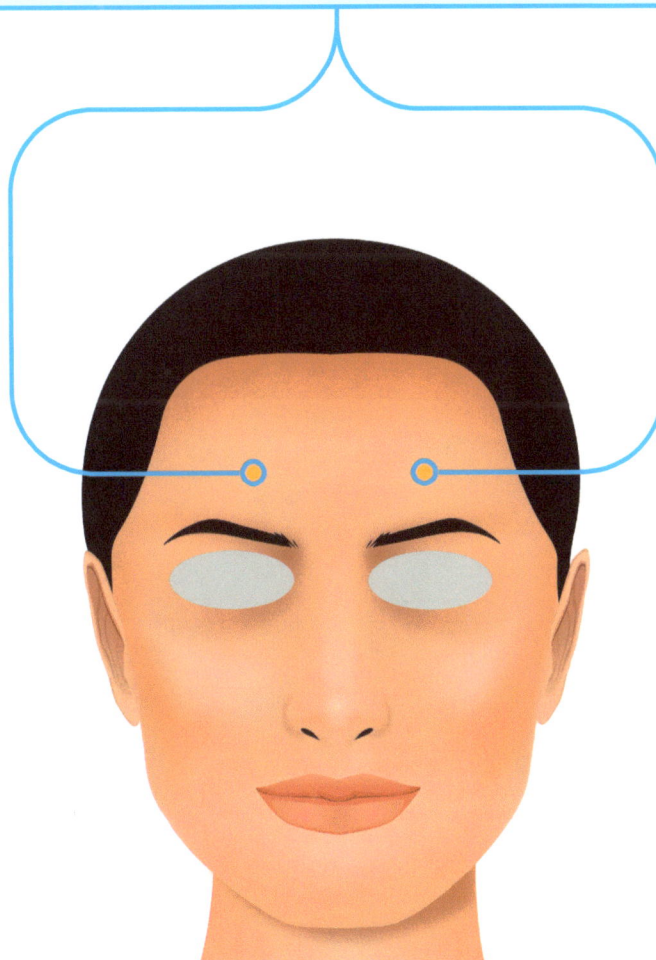

Ear relief

Location: Directly in front of the tragus

Function: Clears heat and stagnation from the ear. Calms the nafs.

Indications: Ear problems of any cause, inflammation of the ear, acute deafness, tinnitus, acute hearing loss.
TMJ, toothache.
Calms the nafs - manic behavior, epilepsy, sensation of pressure below the heart.

Method: A very small cup can be used or drops of blood can be squeezed depending on the nature of the illness as per the other points on the face. This is also a point that can treat mental illness of affectation by sihr or jinn when used in combination with ruqya and other points

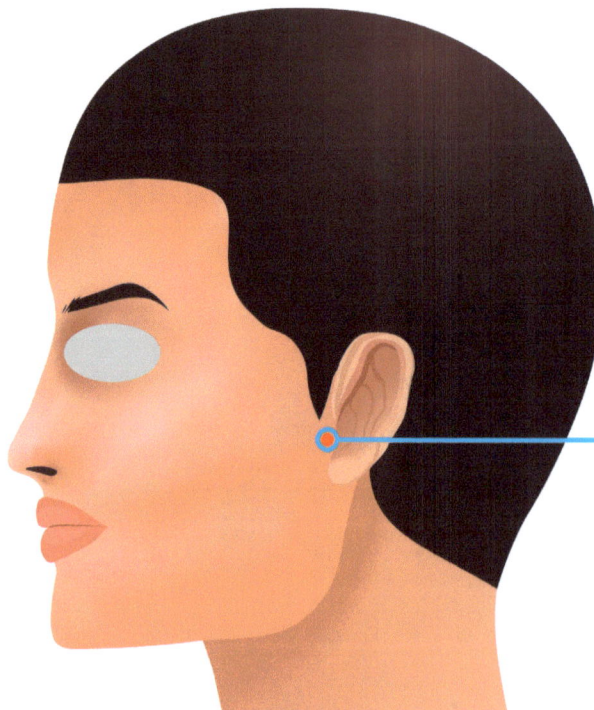

Clear the eyes

Location: In a depression approximately 1 finger breadth below the border of the eyelid directly in line with the pupil of the eye.

Function: Release heat from the eyes

Indications: Eye infections, red, painful and/or itchy eyes, excessive lacrimation, twitching of the eyelids.

Method: (This Hijama point should only be attempted by experienced and properly trained practitioners) Use a surgical blade to make a very small incision, alternatively a single lancet device can be used to make a single incision. Thereafter blood should be allowed to release freely from the point or a small cylindrical cup can be used to remove 10 to 20 drops of blood.

Caution: Only use this point if you are experienced and preferably if you have been trained to use this point.

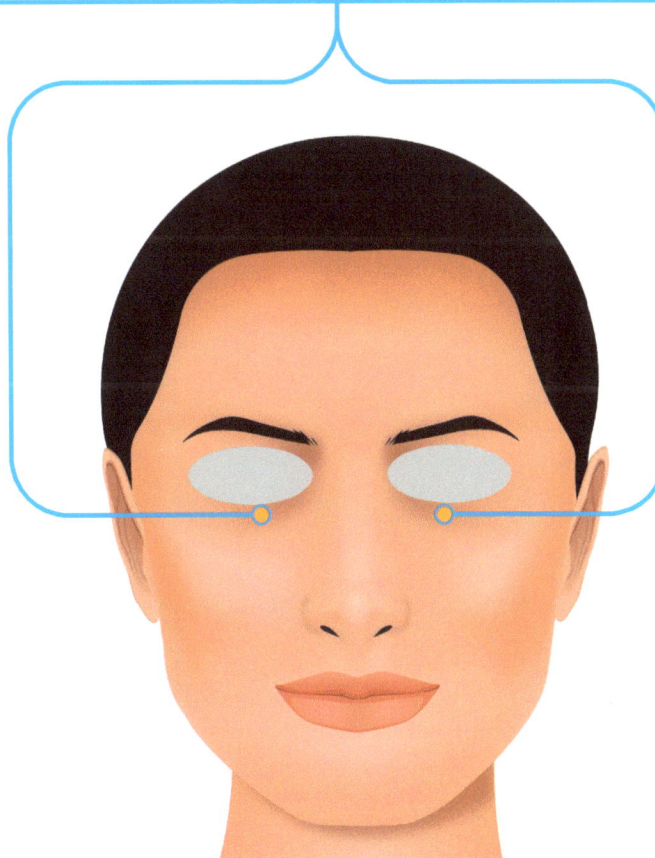

Focus point

Location: Midway between the medial ends of the eyebrows

Function: Balances left and right brain activity, releases heat from the mind, clears stasis.

Indications: Calms the mind - treats insomnia, anxiety, stress. Treats frontal headache and sinus issues - congestion, sinusitis.

Method: Pinch the skin up and use a small blade or lancet to make one incision only, thereafter squeeze drops of blood or place a small cylindrical cup with light pressure. Squeezing is better for this point as often the cup will create pressure around the area and restrict blood flowing to the point. Using a cup will also leave a mark on the face which is undesirable.

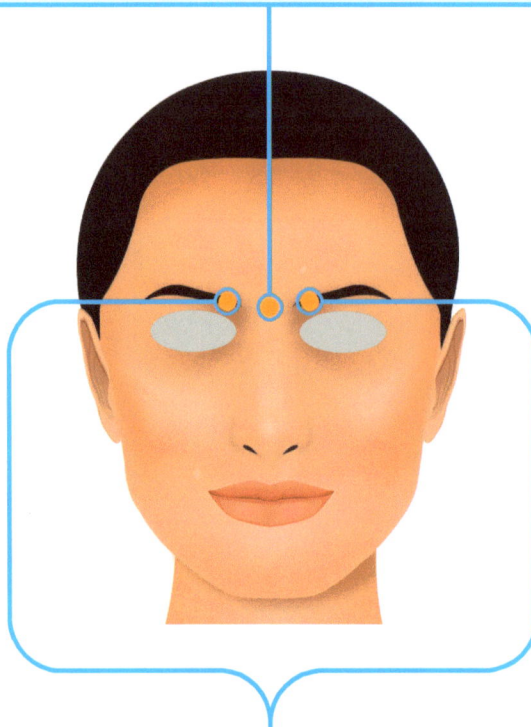

Eye corner

Location: On the medial end of the eyebrow, directly above the inner canthus of the eye (on the supraorbital notch).

Function: Clears heat from the eye and sinuses

Indications: sinus congestion a/or sinus headache. Red, itchy, watery eyes, glaucoma, night blindness, blurry and/or weak vision.

Method: Pinch the skin up and pierce with a lancet or make a very small incision with a blade. Then squeeze 10 to 20 drops of blood.

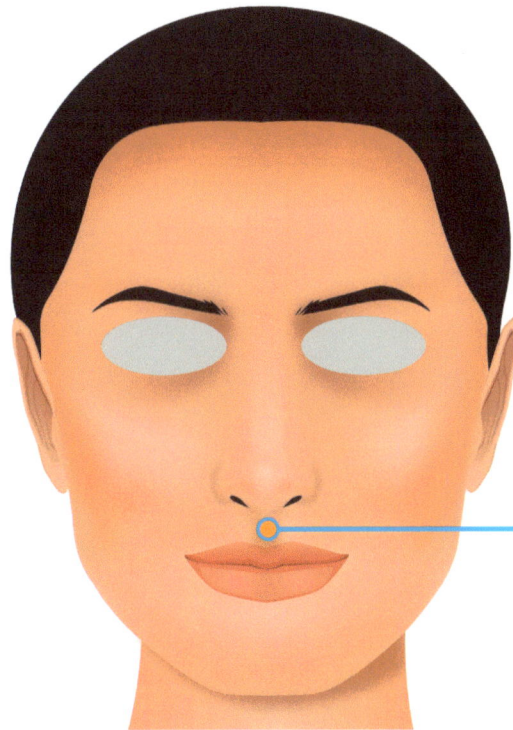

Revive consciousness

Location: At the junction of the upper and middle third of the philtrum.

Function: Revives and restores consciousness and mental function

Indication: Restores consciousness, for shock, revival from fainting, weakness, helps patient to awaken. Also used for acute low back sprain, helps relieve pain and restore motion

Method: Pinch the skin and use a lancet to make multiple incisions. Squeeze to bleed, use strong force and bleed 15 to 20 drops.

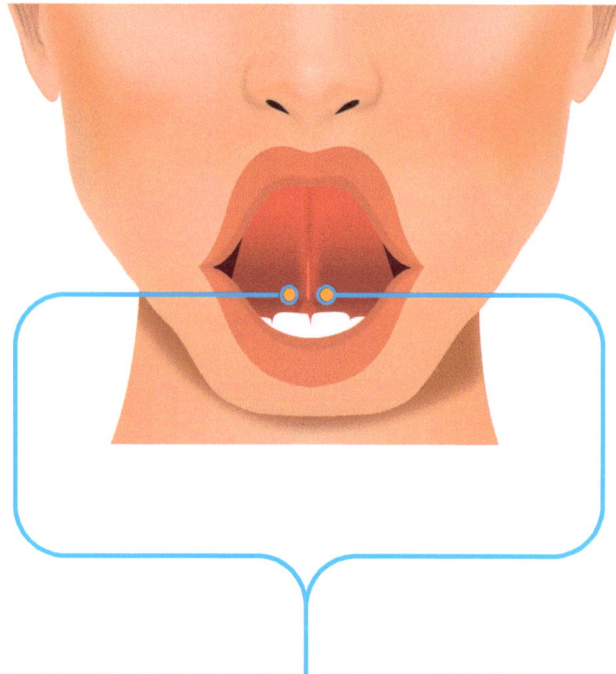

Two veins

Location: The two veins located underneath the tongue

Functions: Moves blood, restores speech, treats toxins, removes heat and wind

Indications: swollen tongue esp. w/difficult speaking, salivary gland issues, post-stroke aphasia.

Method: Hold the patients tongue with a cloth and examine the veins underneath, if they are engorged and purplish then prick each with a surgical blade or lancet.

Caution: Only attempt this treatment if you have been trained and practiced under appropriate supervision.

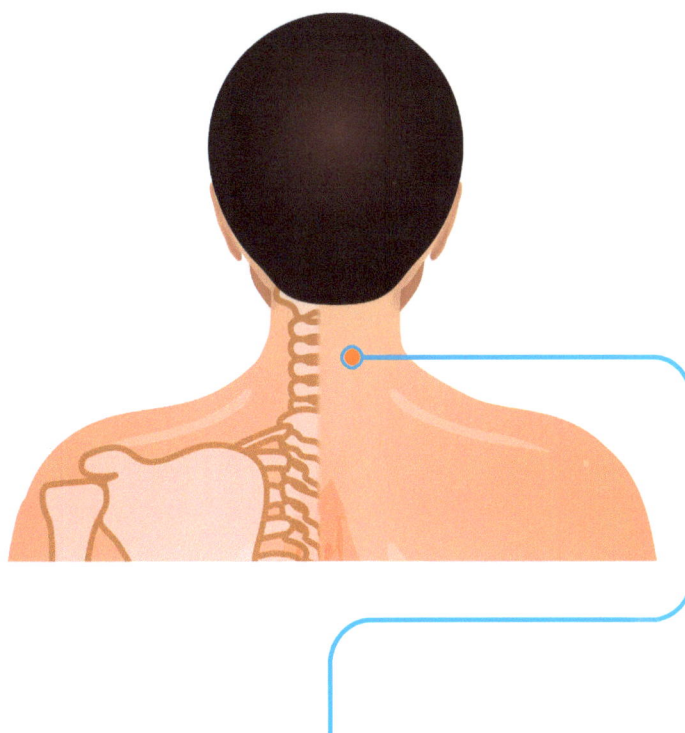

Neck wind

Location: 3 finger breadths above the space between the c7 and t1 palpable protrusions of their spinous processes and 1 finger breadth lateral.

Functions: Relieves local qudra and blood stagnation and stasis, Relieves pain. Can also relieve heat from the lung:

Indications: Lung issues - cough, dyspnea, asthma. Local point for stiff neck, shoulder a/or back pain.

Method: As this point is located on the neck caution should be exercised. Multiple lancet piercings or incisions with a blade may be used with the application of a small to medium cup.

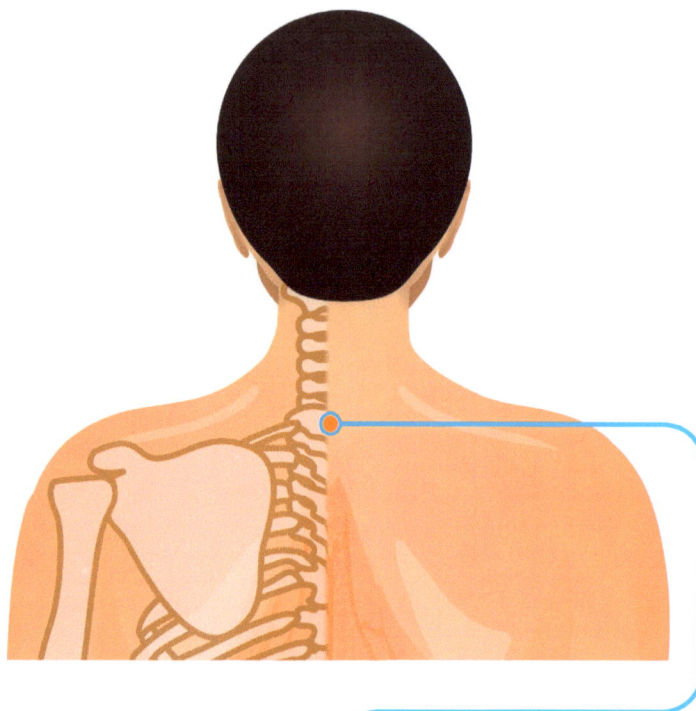

كاهل اول (Kaahil Awwal)

Location: Between the spinous processes of C7 and T1. To locate this point find the most significant protrusion at the junction of the neck and upper back, it will be below this protrusion. It will be on the level of the midpoint of the shoulders.

Functions and Indications: This general area (which includes the area between the shoulder blades and extending from this point downwards) is one of the 9 "sunnah" areas that were used by the Prophet ﷺ in Hijama. Kaahil Awwal is a very important point in the body for different types of therapies and illnesses. it can be used to drain excess (heat) from the body or even to address weakness and cold of the body by applying heat therapies (see the courses page for more information on heat therapies)

Excess heat conditions include febrile disease (fevers), malaria, hot blood diseases, neck pain and rigidity, back stiffness, psychosis, epilepsy, seizures, pneumonia, schizophrenia, bronchitis, asthma, hepatitis and eczema. Also heat in the lungs, and labored breathing with yellow mucus as in the case of pneumonia.

Method: This point can be bled with a medium to large cup with multiple incisions either with a lancet or surgical blade.

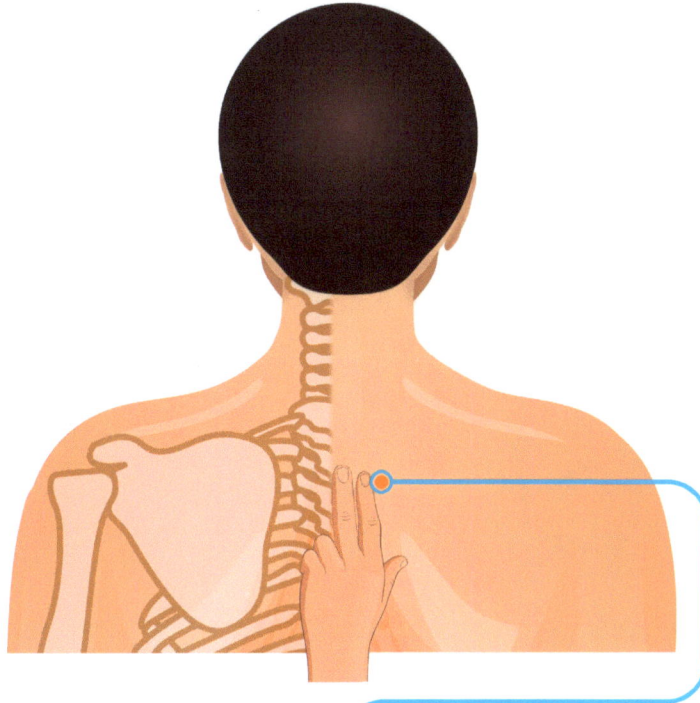

كاهل ثاني (Kaahil Thaani)

Location: 2 fingers lateral to the spinous process of T3

Functions: Release heat from the lungs

Indications: cough, asthma, bronchitis, sore throat, nasal congestion, shortness of breath, weakness of the voice, consumption, steaming bone disorder, also useful for skin disorders, itching, acne, hives, etc.

Method: This point can be bled with a medium to large cup with multiple incisions either with a lancet or surgical blade.

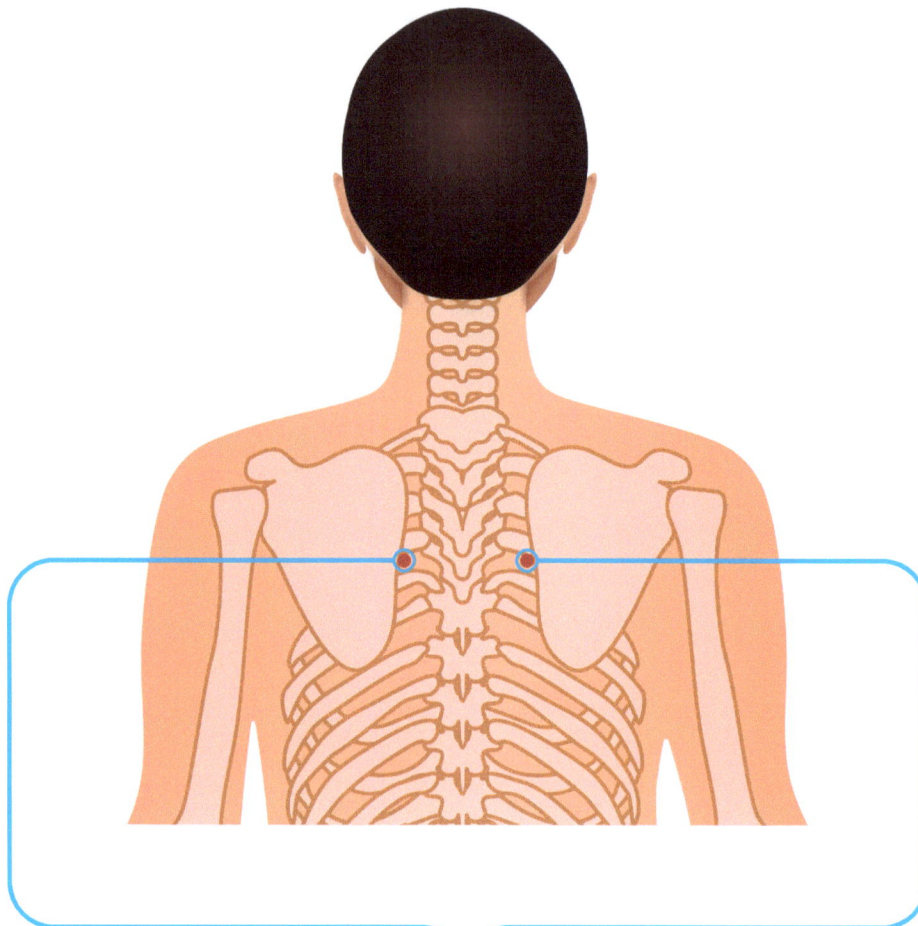

كاهل ثالث (Kaahil Thaalith)

Location: 4 finger lateral to the spinous process of T4

Functions: Treats chronic heat in the lungs

Indications: Main point for all disorders of the Lung, asthma, dyspnea, cough, tuberculosis, etc

Method: This point can be bled with a medium to large cup with multiple incisions either with a lancet or surgical blade.

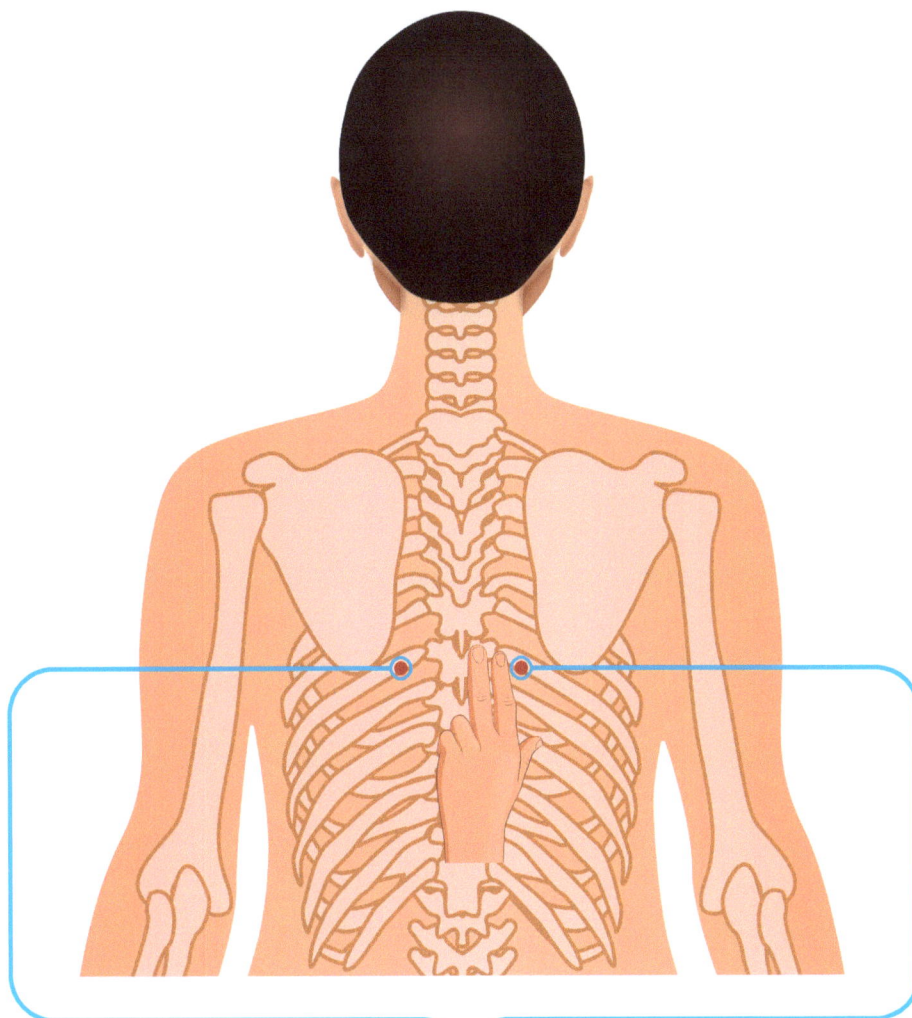

Back Blood point

Location: Two fingers lateral to the spinous process of T7

Function: Treats diseases of the blood due to heat and/or stasis

Indications: coughing or vomiting of blood, blood in the stool, menstrual problems due to heat and stasis such as excessive bright red bleeding, spotting due to heat, amenorrhea due to stasis. Important point for red, itchy skin disorders, from heat in the blood such as eczema, carbuncles, also treats manic depression and can also assist with vomiting, epigastric pain, reflux.

Method: This point can be bled with a medium to large cup with multiple incisions either with a lancet or surgical blade.

Comment: This point as well as the Kaahil points can be used for general Hijama to remove toxins from the blood. This should be done based on the climate and the constitution of the patient.

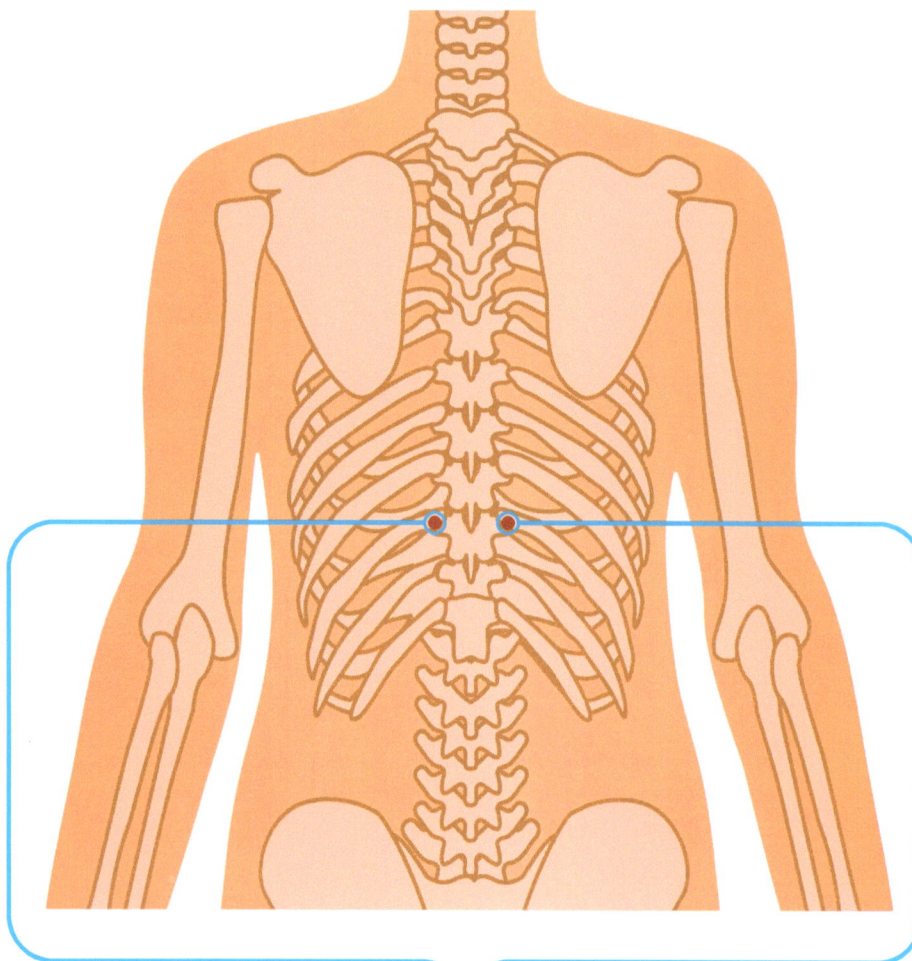

Liver point

Location: Two fingers lateral to the spine at the level of T9

Functions: Clears heat and blood stasis from the liver

Indications: This is the main point for all Liver related heat or excess blood (stagnant) conditions whether physical or emotional (anger, frustration, irritability, short temper)
Used for - hepatitis, jaundice, cirrhosis.
Brightens the eyes - important point for eye problems, pain, itching, dryness, redness, blurred vision, visual dizziness, twitching, night blindness. Useful for hypochondriac a/or subcostal pain/distention. Can also treat menstrual problems due to heat or stagnation. Note that bleeding this point is not useful for dryness of the liver (blood deficiency of the liver) or diseases due to dryness.

Method: This point can be bled with a medium to large cup with multiple incisions either with a lancet or surgical blade.

Shoulder tension point

Location: On the shoulder directly above the nipple at the midpoint of a line connecting T7 and the acromion at the highest point of the shoulder.

Function and Indication: This is a local point for occipital headache, tight trapezius muscles and neck or shoulder pain.
Can also be used to treat mastitis and breast abscesses.

Method: This point can be bled with a medium to large cup with multiple incisions either with a lancet or surgical blade.

Contraindicated: Do not use during pregnancy, can cause miscarriage. (Hijama should be avoided in pregnancy in general as there is a great need for blood to nourish the fetus)

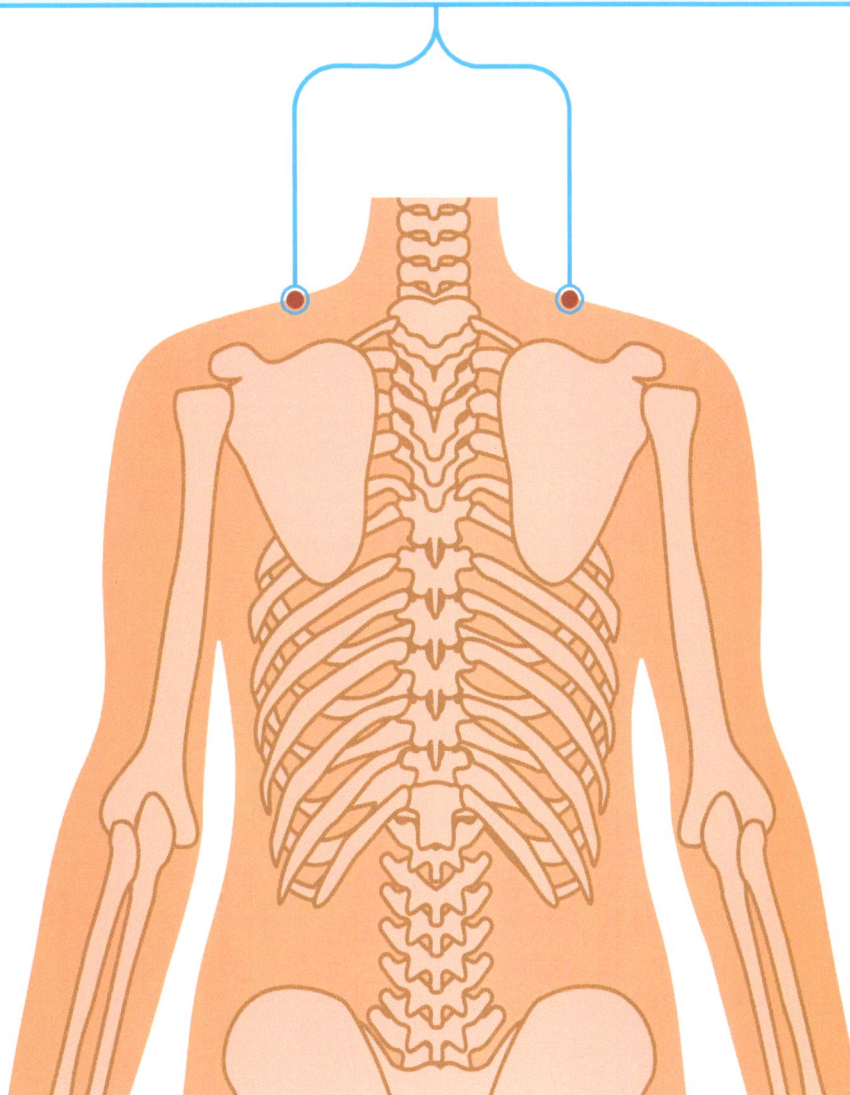

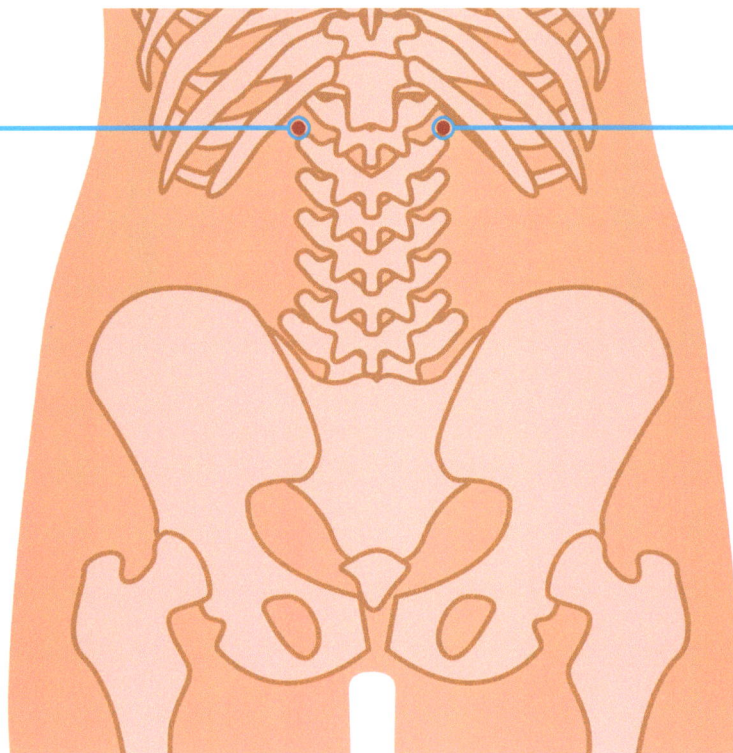

Stomach point

Location: 2 fingers lateral to the spine at the level of T12

Functions: Clears heat from the stomach

Indications: Main point for all Stomach related issues, harmonizes the stomach, transforms damp and resolves stagnation: food stagnation, abdominal distention, borborygmus, mouth ulcers, vomiting, belching, nausea, etc. Can also treat facial acne due to stomach heat, constipation due to stomach heat.

Method: This point can be bled with a medium to large cup with multiple incisions either with a lancet or surgical blade.

Heart disease point

Location: 2 finger breadths lateral to the spine, level with T5.

Functions and Indications: For all stagnation and excess heart conditions: palpitations, anxiety, stress, etc.
Also treats liver conditions such as stagnation of Liver qudra resulting in depression, anxiety, panic attacks, etc.
This point can be used after a heart attack with a small cup as it has been proven to improve healing after. Allow 2 weeks between sessions. Only use in excess conditions however and assess the strength of the patient before doing so. Also ensure that the patient is not taking any anti-coagulant medication (blood thinners) such as warfarin etc.

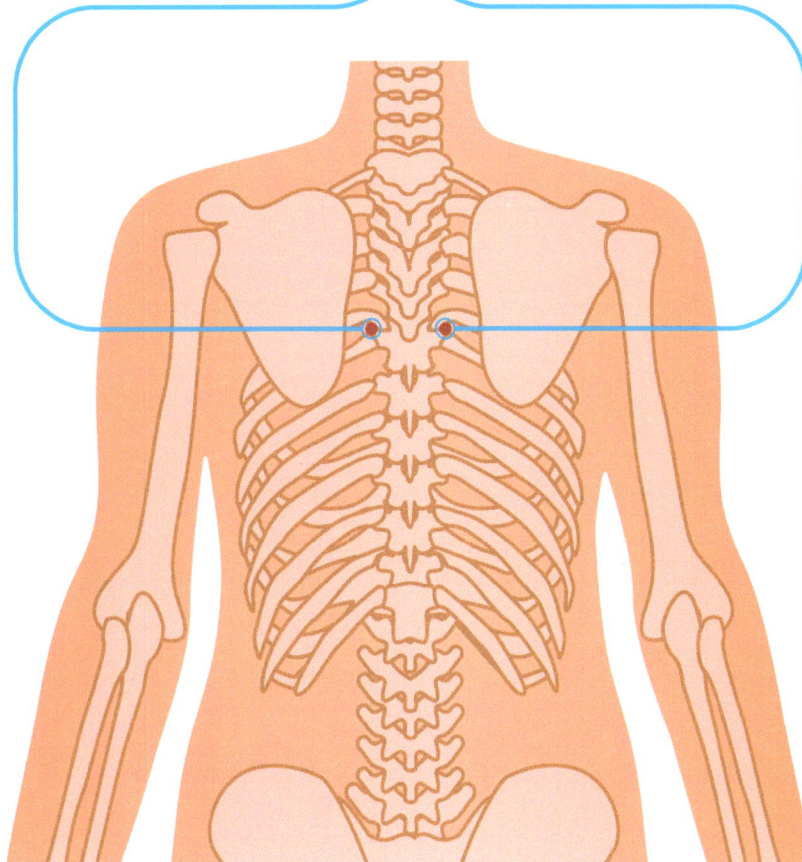

Gallbladder point

Location: 2 fingerbreadths lateral to the spine, level with T10.

Functions and Indications: Treats alternating fever and chills. Main point for damp heat in the Liver and Gall Bladder: hepatitis, cholecystitis, jaundice, vomiting, flank pain and distension, bitter taste in the mouth. Often combined with the Liver connection point. Pain along the sides of the body from any etiology, intercostal neuralgia, rib pain, trauma, herpes zoster. insomnia, anxiety (often with bitter taste in the mouth), palpitations.

Method: Make 3 to 5 small incisions with a surgical blade or lancets and apply a small to medium cup to draw blood.

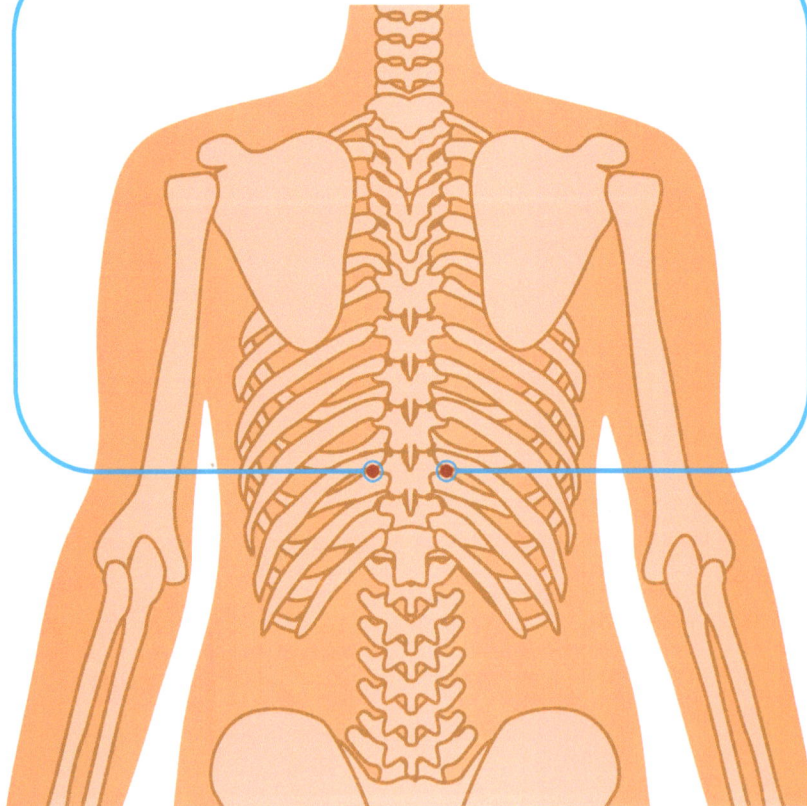

Upper back malaria point

Location: On the midline of the spine, below T1.

Functions and Indications: Treats inflammatory diseases affecting the bones, chills and fever.
Important point for malaria.
Stiffness of the neck a/or spine, heavy head, headaches.

Method: This point is very sensitive to bleeding and is therefore only used in acute emergency cases. It is bled with a lancet or surgical blade without a cup being applied. Between 2 to 5 drops of blood are squeezed out after making the incision.

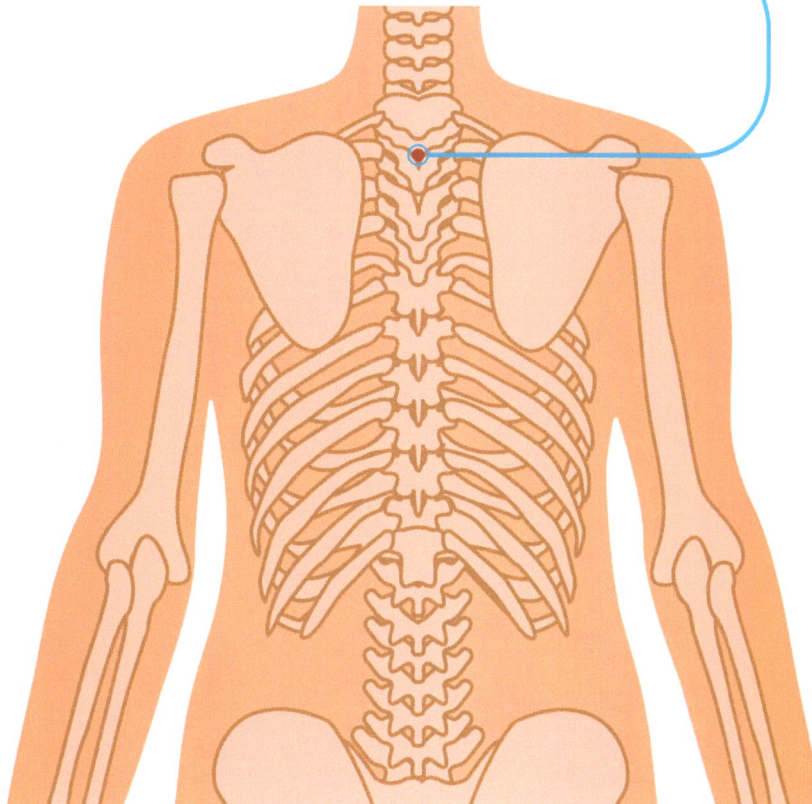

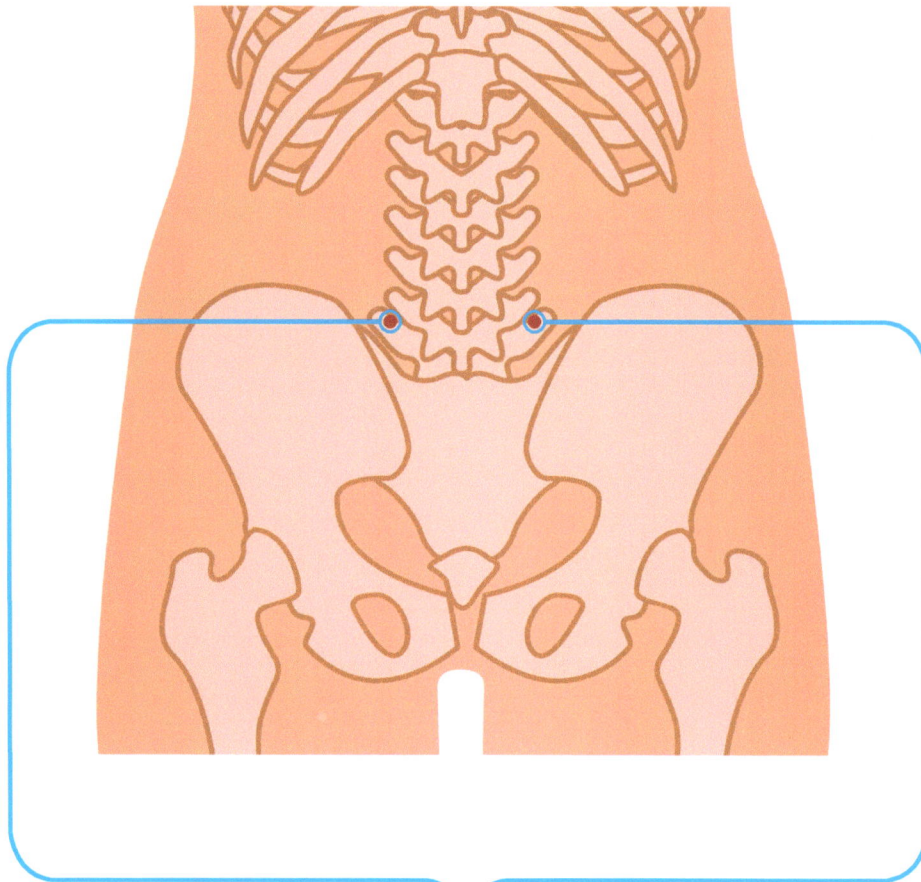

Colon point

Location: 2 fingers lateral to the spine at the level of L4

Functions: Clears heat from the colon and local area. Moves blood in the local area

Indications: Treats constipation, diarrhea, dysentery, colitis, IBS due to heat or stasis. Also treats lower back pain when associated with constipation and/or menstrual problems due to stagnation or heat.

Method: This point can be bled with a medium to large cup with multiple incisions either with a lancet or surgical blade.

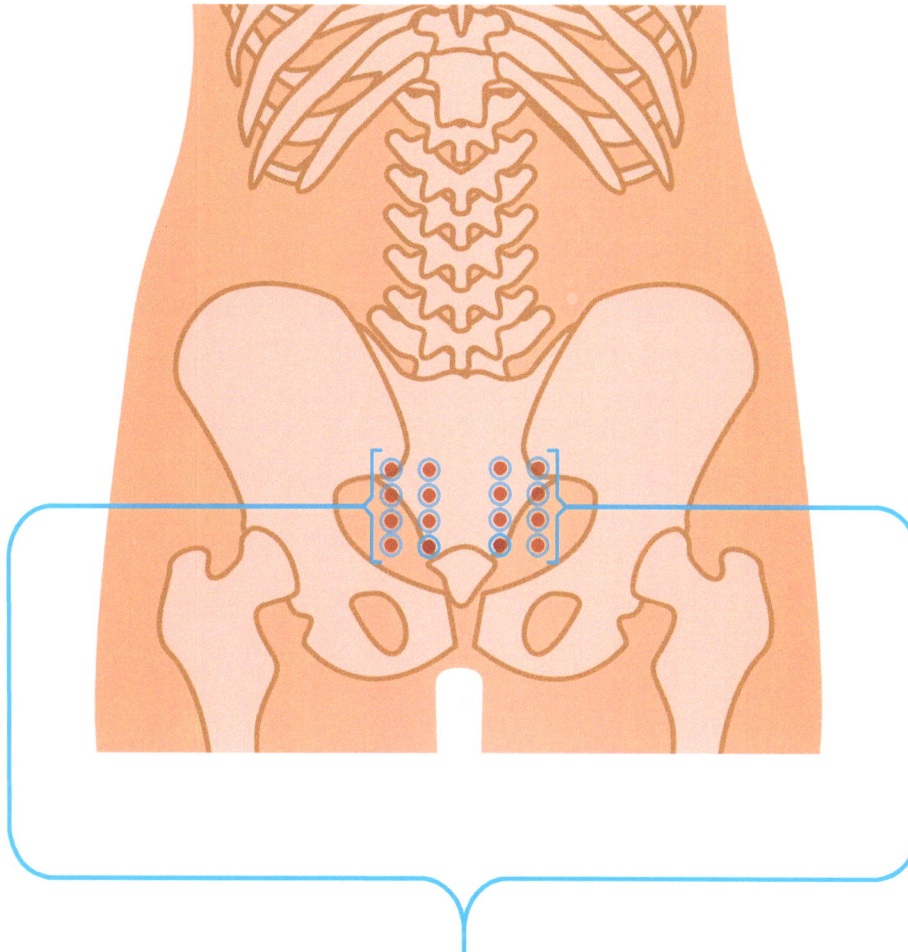

Sacral region

Location: This area lies over the sacrum

Functions & Indications: This is a general area that is bled for many problems including menstrual problems, infertility, lower back pain etc that is either due to heat in these organs or due to stagnation of blood.

Method: Check for blue or purple veins in the area. If found this is an indication that blood is stagnant in the area. Choose a place directly over the center of the sacrum and administer Hijama to the area with a small to medium cup. Repeat the procedure once a month or every second month and combine with dietary and herbal therapy as necessary.

Back pain point

Location: In the depression approximately 5 fingers lateral to the spine at the level of L4

Functions: Treats lower back pain due to multiple causes.

Indications: For excess type back pain that is characterised by sharp and stabbing pain that restricts movement and may also be associated with spider veins in the region

Method: Make incisions and apply a medium cup. In patients with a strong constitution a large cup can be used. if there is associated kidney weakness use a heating therapy in addition.

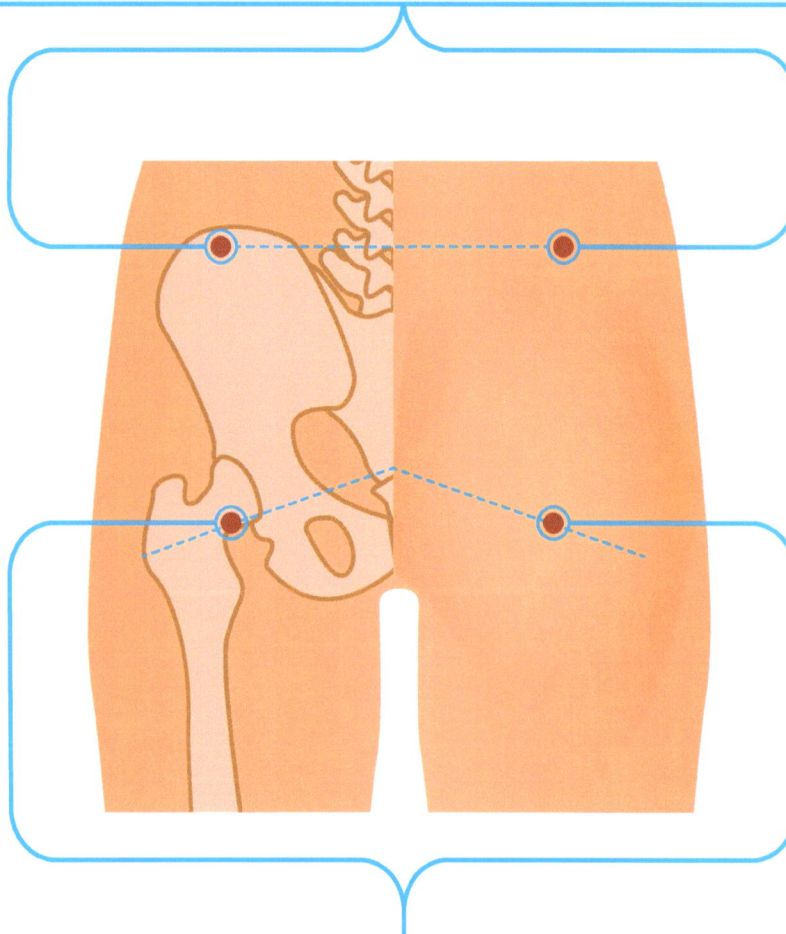

Sciatica point

Location: At the junction of the lateral 1/3 and medial 2/3 distance between the prominence of the greater trochanter and the hiatus of the sacrum, (located with the patient in a lateral recumbent position with thigh flexed).

Functions and indications: Treats sciatic type pain

Method: First apply the cup without bleeding for 7 to 10 minutes to draw blood from the deep section of this point. Thereafter make incisions and bleed a medium to large cup if the patient is strong, or a small cup in a weak patient.

Rear shoulder

Location: 1 finger above the posterior end of the axillary fold, posterior and inferior to the shoulder joint, found with the arm adducted.

Function and Indications: Local point for shoulder and arm pain and/or movement/control issues. Motor control issues of the hand.

Method: This point can be bled with a medium to large cup with multiple incisions either with a lancet or surgical blade.

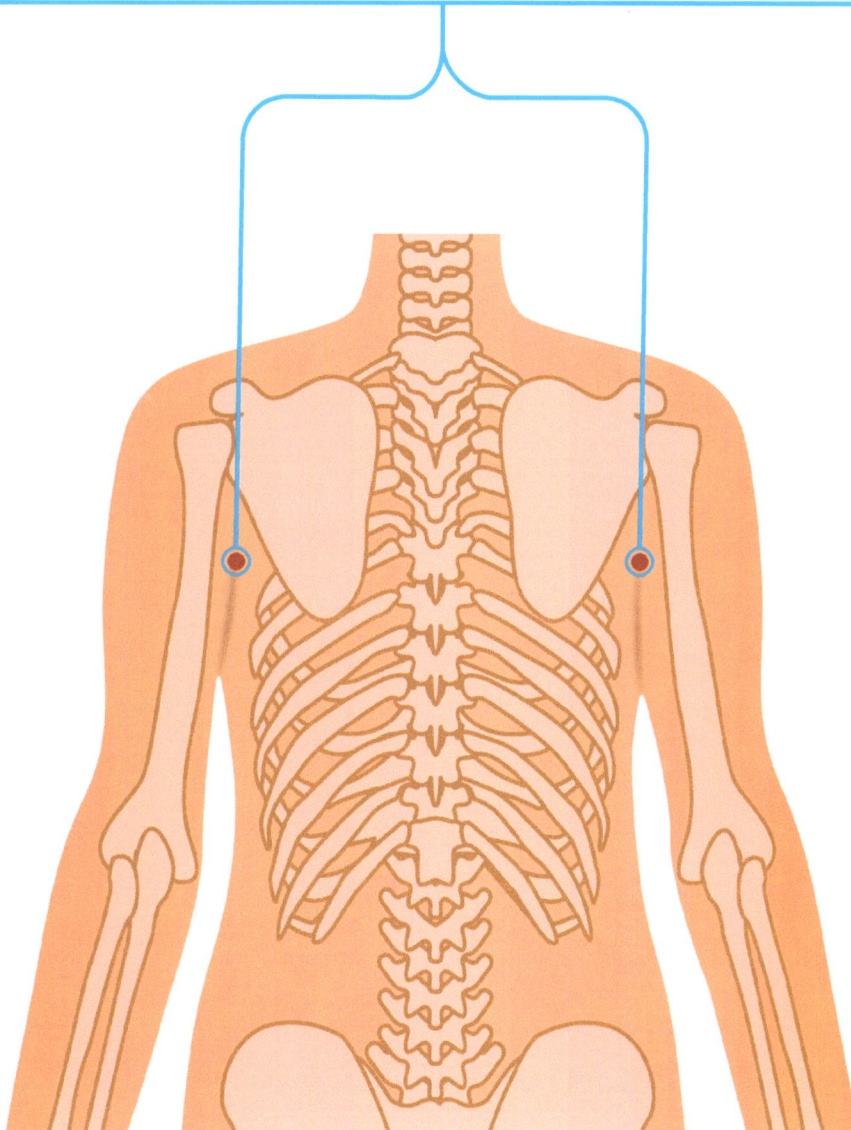

Revive respiration

Location: On the radial side of the thumb, 2mm lateral and superior to the corner of the nail.

Functions: Clears heat from the lung and throat. Arouses the brain and settles the nafs.

Indications: Sore throat due to heat and toxins (tonsillitis), cough with blood due to heat, nosebleed due to heat, high fever. Can also be used due to drug reaction causing delirium or unconsciousness.

Method: Bleed with a surgical blade or lancet and allow blood to flow freely or squeeze 10 drops or more.

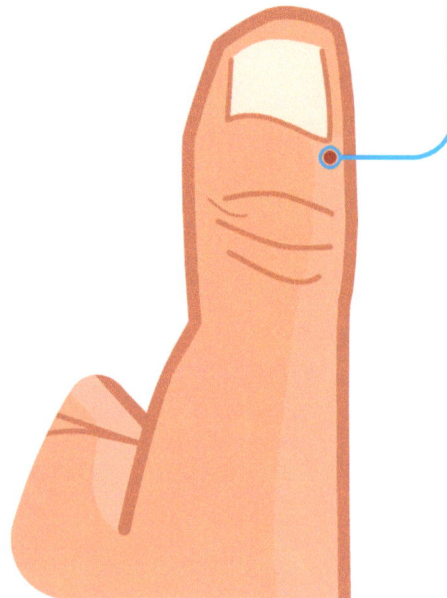

Brain release point

Location: This point is located at the tip of the middle finger.

Functions: It can be bled 3 to 7 drops of blood for cases of extreme heat affecting the brain (and heart) characterised by sudden stroke, convulsions and speech disorders together with heat signs such as red face. This point can also be used for restoring consciousness

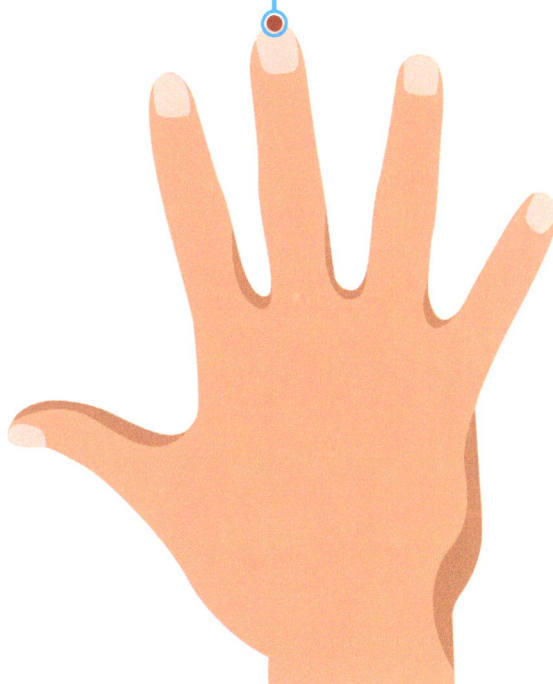

Master of the face

Location: On the dorsum of the hand between the 1st and 2nd metacarpals approximately 1/2 way up the lateral edge of the 2nd metacarpal

Function: Clears heat infection from the upper respiratory tract. Treats pain and depression of qudra. Treats facial disorders.

Indications: Headache, toothache, sore throat, red eyes, swollen eyes due to allergy, goiter, tmj problems.

Method: Make 2 to 3 incisions with a surgical blade or lancet and use a small cylindrical cup to draw blood. Do not use this point during pregnancy

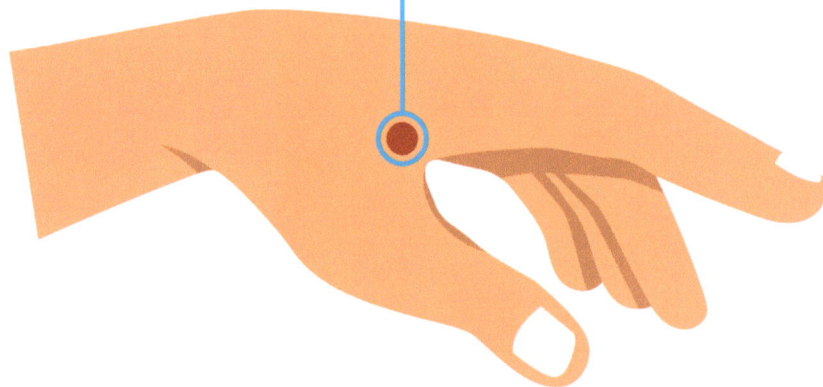

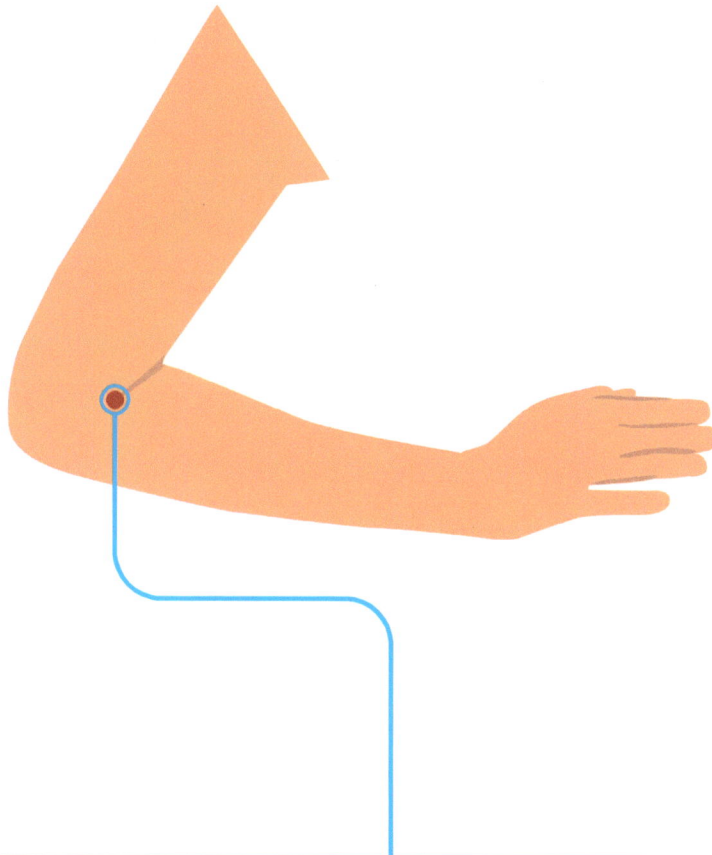

Skin cleanse

Location: When the elbow is flexed, this Hijama point is in the depression at the lateral end of the crease.

Function: Clears heat and toxins from the skin and colon

Indications: Clears heat from the skin, colon and lungs. Cools the blood. Treats fever, high blood pressure, urticaria.

Method: Make a few incisions with a surgical blade or lancets and use a small to medium cup to draw blood from the area.

Shoulder side

Location: Anterior and inferior to the acromion in the anterior depression when the arm is abducted.

Function: Treats blood stasis in the shoulder area

Indications: Shoulder pain

Method: First apply a cup to draw blood to the area, massaging towards the cup while it is on. Leave on for a few minutes monitoring the color of the skin, when it turns a bit red, remove and make 3 to 5 incisions with a surgical blade or lancet. Then apply a small to medium cup and draw blood. Repeat this procedure once a week or once a fortnight. (This is why you should only draw a small to medium cup of blood in one session)

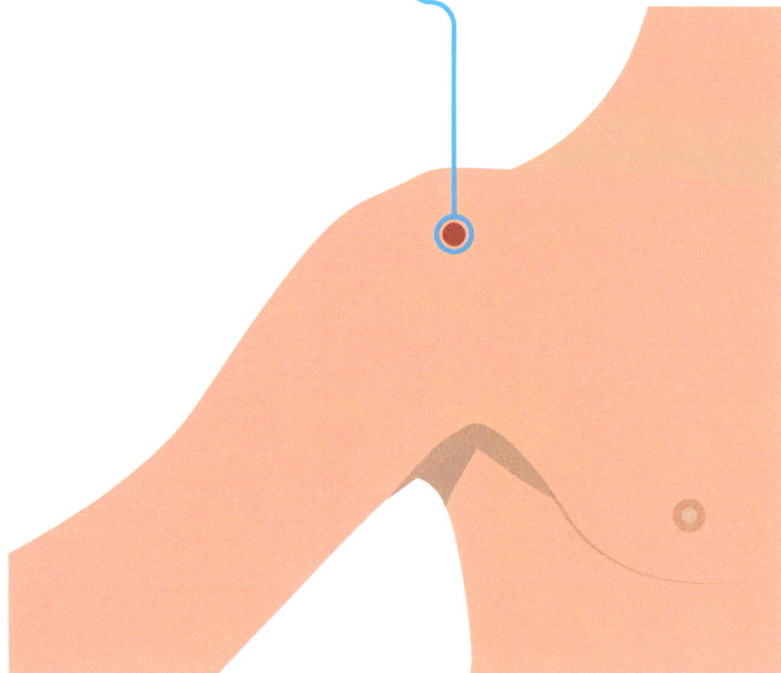

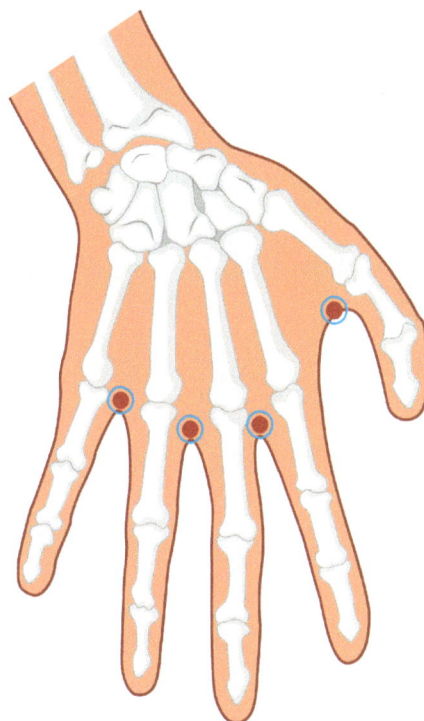

Hand malaria points

Location: On the dorsum of the hand, at the webs between each finger, at the junction of the red & white skin.

Functions: Treats malaria and malaria type fevers

Method: Bleed each point with a lancet or surgical blade and allow to bleed.

Heart connection

Location: 1/4 way inferior on the line drawn from the bottom of the sternum to the umbilicus

Functions and Indications: Use only for excess conditions characterised by fire (in terms of Traditional Islamic Medicine Diagnosis) Treats angina, pain/tightness in the Heart area.
Nausea, reflux, acid regurgitation, vomiting, abdominal a/or epigastric pain.
Mental disturbances such as manic depression, muddled thinking, anger outbursts.

Method: This is not a commonly used point, however it is to be considered if there is a connection with digestive disturbance and mental/heart related issues, one example is a patient who has a very large appetite and also suffers from mania, high temper etc. This point can then be used after first trying the general points on the back.

Use a small cup for the first treatment after making 3 to 5 incisions with a surgical blade or lancet.

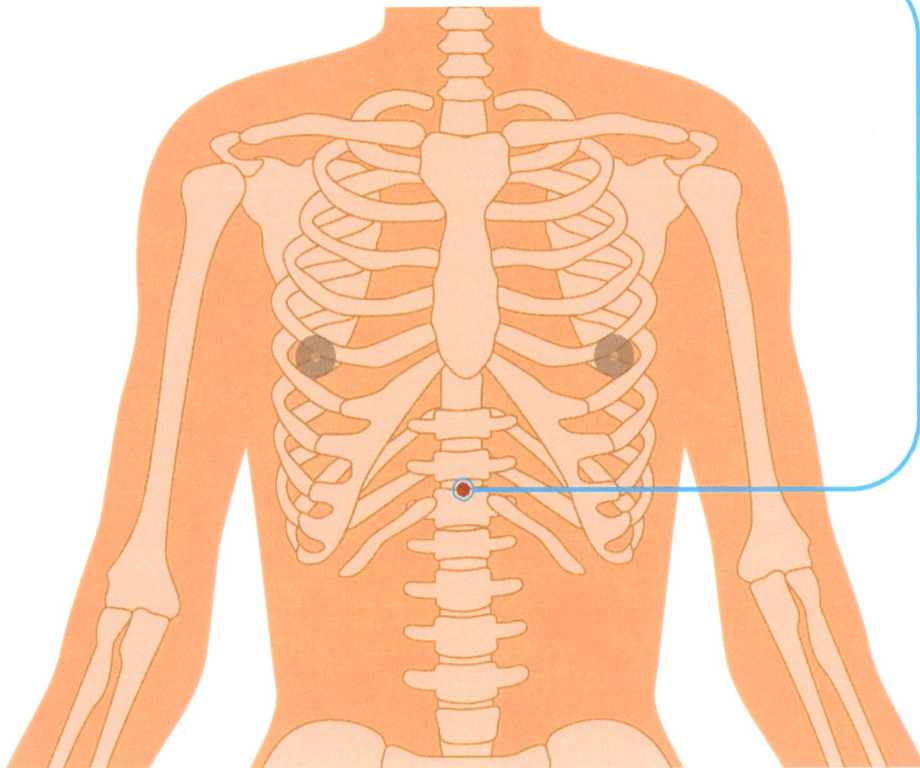

Stomach connection

Location: Midway between the bottom of the sternum and the umbilicus

Functions and Indications: Excess (heat) stomach disorders causing pain, bloating, reflux, vomiting, diarrhea, jaundice.

Method: Use a small cup after making 3 to 5 incisions with a surgical blade or lancet

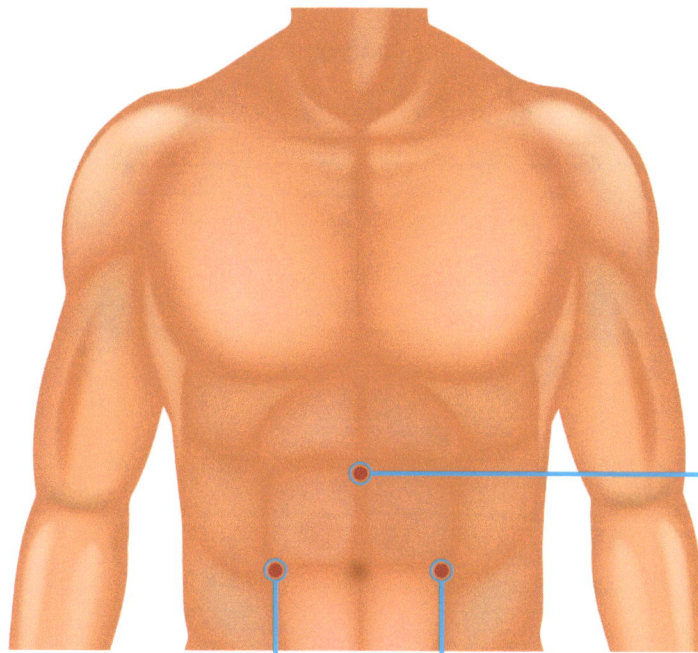

Colon connection

Location: 3 fingers lateral to the umbilicus

Functions and indications: Treats all intestinal issues due to excess heat or stasis of blood - constipation, diarrhea, dysentary, distention, pain, masses/accumulations of any type.
Irregular menstruation, painful menstruation, fibroids/cysts, fertility issues and leukorrhea.

Method: Use a small to medium cup after making 3 to 5 incisions with a surgical blade or lancet. (this is a sensitive area and care should be taken, do not draw blood excessively in women and those suffering from anaemia)

Breast excess

Location: This point is located underneath the breast directly below the nipple, in the fifth intercostal space.

Functions and Indications: Any issues due to excess with the breasts - mastitis, pain/swelling, insufficient lactation. If the issue is due to deficiency, then do not bleed but rather apply dry cupping.

Method: This point should only be used by a female practitioner for a female patient. Take precautions as it is a sensitive area and only use if necessary. Make 3 small incisions with a surgical blade or lancet (preferred) and use a small cup to draw blood. This is only for cases of excess which will be characterised by inflammation.

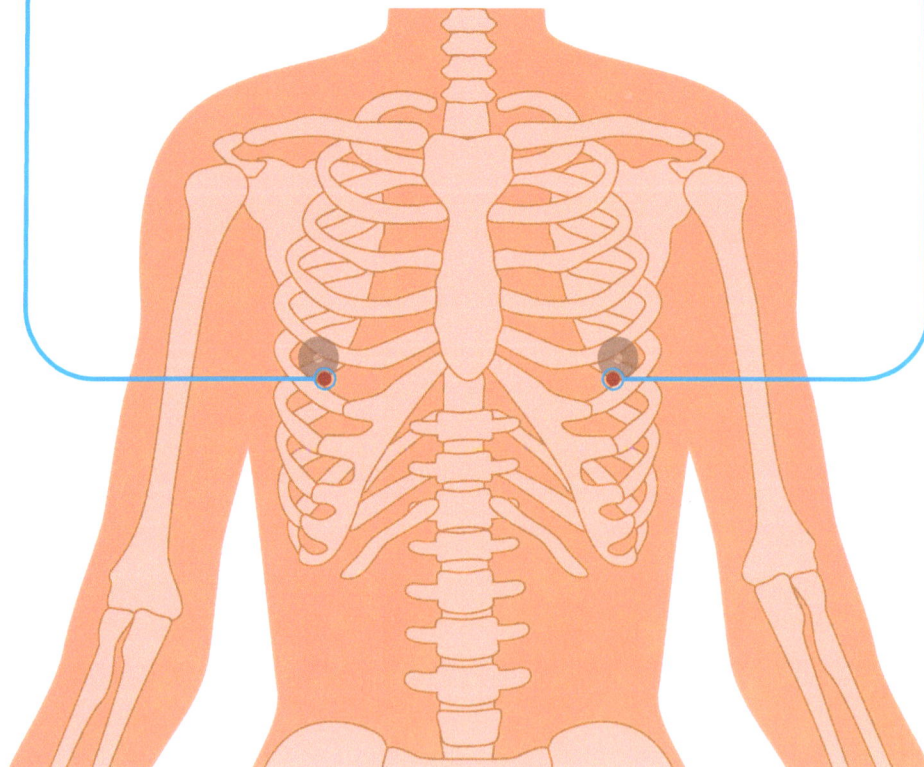

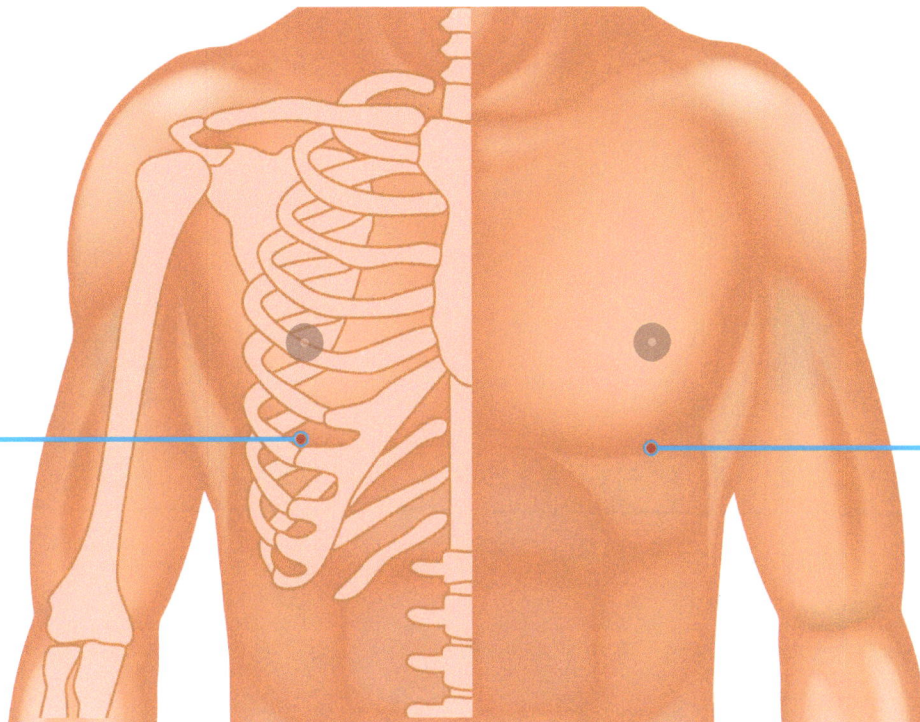

Liver connection

Location: Directly below the nipple, (5 fingers lateral to the midline) in the 6th intercostal space. This point is normally tender in those who have liver diseases or stress, anger and frustration issues. Also in those who suffer from PMS and other menstrual illnesses due to qudra stagnation.

Functions and indications: Releases heat and accumulation from the liver. Treats subcostal tension, chest/rib pain, Liver overacting on the Lung causing cough and shortness of breath (this usually occurs as a response to stress) also treats blood stagnation causing hepatitis, gallstones. Also used for excess related anger and irritability issues and mania due to liver fire. Hijama should not be done for deficiency conditions of the liver, do dry cupping instead

Method: Make 3 to 5 small incisions with a surgical blade or lancets and apply a small to medium cup to draw blood.

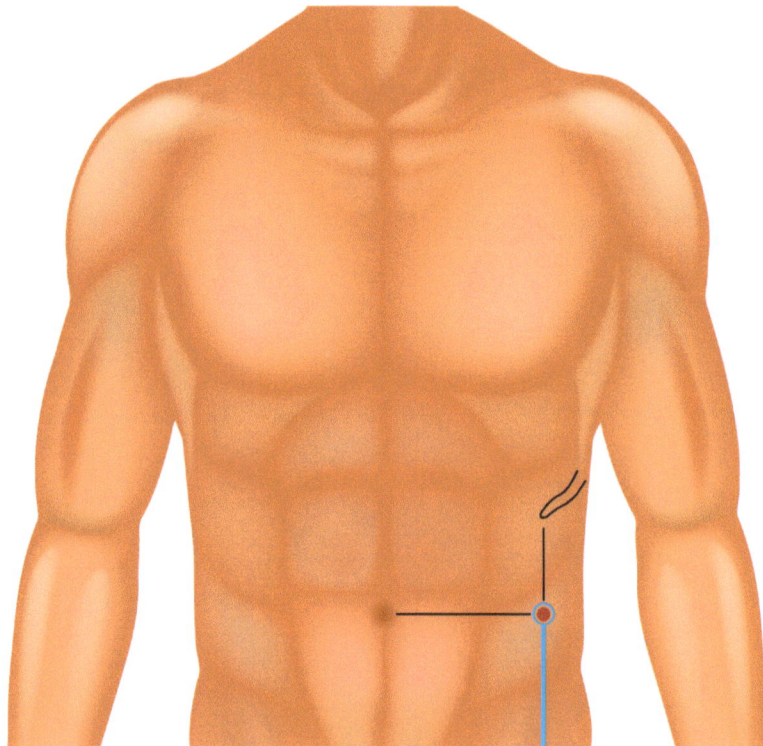

Menstrual regulation

Location: On the lateral side of the abdomen, 2 fingers cun below where the vertical line from the free end of the 11th rib and the horizontal line of the umbilicus intersect.

Functions: This is a useful Hijama point to treat menstrual disorders due to heat or blood stasis although it should be considered after using the other menstrual points. Treats leukorrhea from excess, gynecological disorders due to heat and stasis, blood stasis infertility. Can also treat menstrual related pains, cramping, bloating a/or migraines although with these orders there is always an underlying deficiency that must be diagnosed and treated at the same time.

Method: Make 3 to 5 small incisions with a surgical blade or lancets and apply a small to medium cup to draw blood.

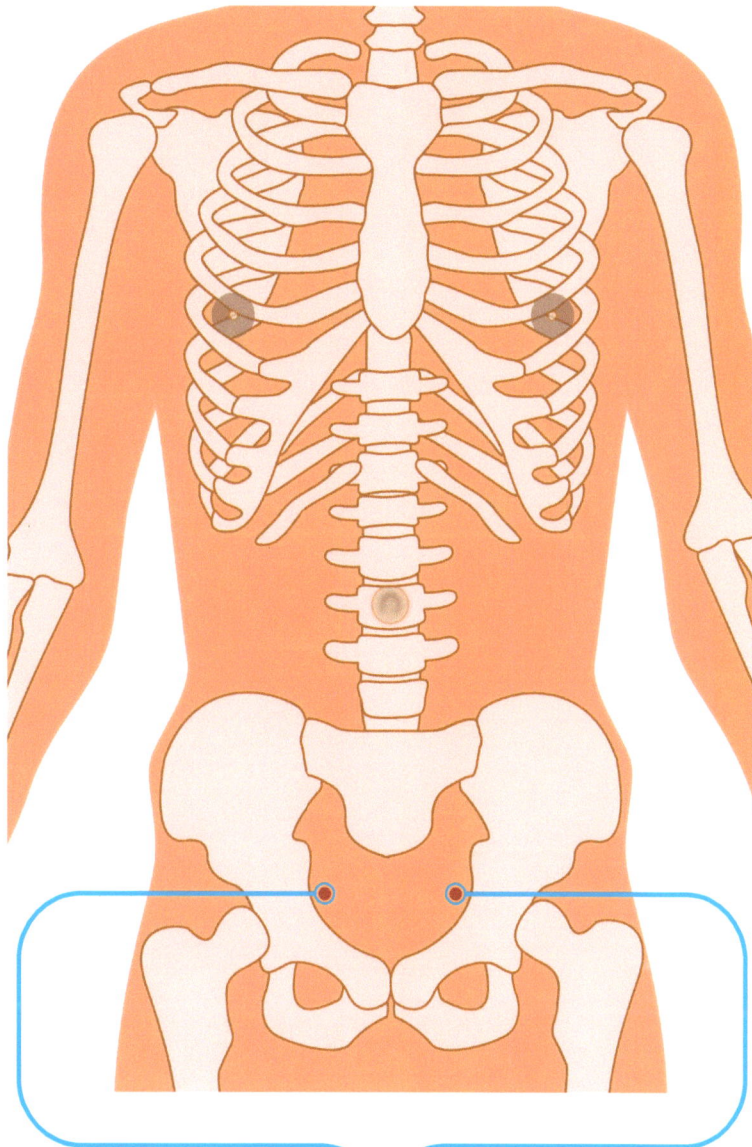

Return menses

Location: 3 fingers lateral to the midline, 5 fingers below the navel

Functions and Indications: This point moves blood in the uterus and is classically known to return menses that have stopped due to a blockage of blood.

Method: Make 3 to 5 small incisions with a lancet or surgical blade and use a small to medium cup to draw blood

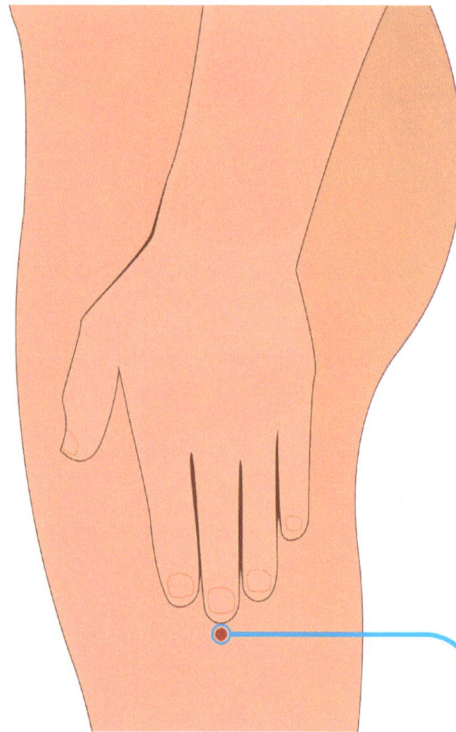

Thigh side point

Location: On the midline of the lateral aspect of the thigh, 2 hand widths above the transverse popliteal crease, another way to locate this point is when the patient is standing erect with hands close to their sides the point is at the tip of their middle finger.

Functions and Indications: Treats lateral and posterior leg issues such as sciatica, weakness, numbness, post-stroke symptoms of lower limbs. Also treats red, itchy, skin disorders from excess factors anywhere on the body. Used often for sciatic nerve issues, lower back pain and leg muscle issues.

Method: For excess conditions or stagnation or those with minor deficiency components a medium to large cup of blood can be drawn (based on the patients constitution). For deficiency conditions apply dry cupping.

Tendons connection

Location: In a depression anterior and inferior to the head of the fibula

Functions and indications: This point is useful for treating tendon and muscle disorders anywhere in the body, including contracture, cramping, pain, spasm, weakness, numbness, paralysis.
Also treats sciatica and issues with the low back, hip, a/or lower limbs, knees.
Also removes excess from the gallbladder such as heat and dampness, therefore can treat cholecystitis, hepatitis, jaundice, nausea, vomiting, bitter taste in mouth, gallstones.
Also useful for the symptoms of alternating chills/fevers, costal pain, bitter taste in mouth which may be due to latent infection that has affected the liver and gallbladder.
Can also treat counterflow qudra flow causing nausea, vomiting, indigestion.

Method: Make 3 small incisions only in the depression area with a lancet or surgical blade and apply a small cup to the area to draw blood. A cylindrical cup can also be used. A large cup may not hold well here depending on the patients surface anatomy.

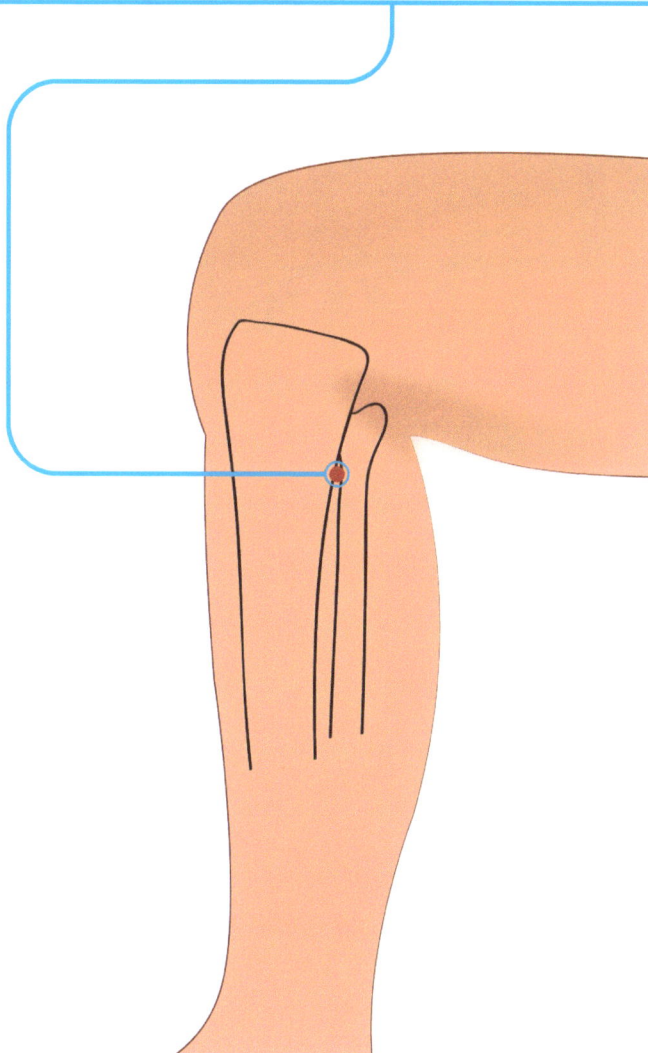

Rabies point

Location: Midway between the lateral malleolus and the previous point (Tendons connection)

Functions: Treats rabies w/rage, fever, convulsions, also treats acute cholecystitis and acute painful skin conditions.

Method: Make 3 small incisions only in the depression area with a lancet or surgical blade and apply a small cup to the area to draw blood. A cylindrical cup can also be used. A large cup may not hold well here depending on the patients surface anatomy.

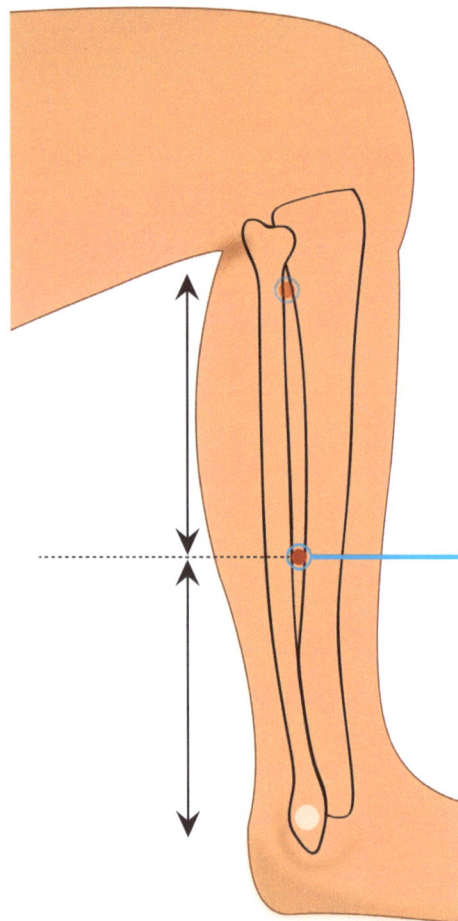

Kabd Thani

Location: This area is located at the web between the big toe and the next toe.

Functions and Indications: It can be bled to treat extreme irritability, red face/eyes/tongue, burning urination and extreme vertex headache.

Method: After making a few small incisions with a lancet or surgical blade, 7 to 10 drops of blood can be squeezed out or a very small cup may also be applied.

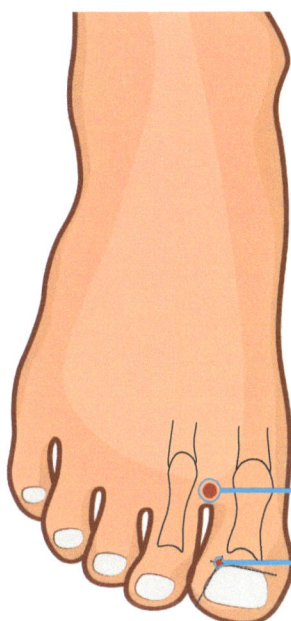

Kabd Awwal

Location: 2mm from the lateral corner of the nail of the big toe.

Functions and indications: it is used for hot types of loss of consciousness, swollen genitals and uterine/menstrual bleeding

Method: This point is very sensitive to bleeding and is therefore only used in acute emergency cases. It is bled with a lancet or surgical blade without a cup being applied. Between 2 to 5 drops of blood are squeezed out after making the incision.

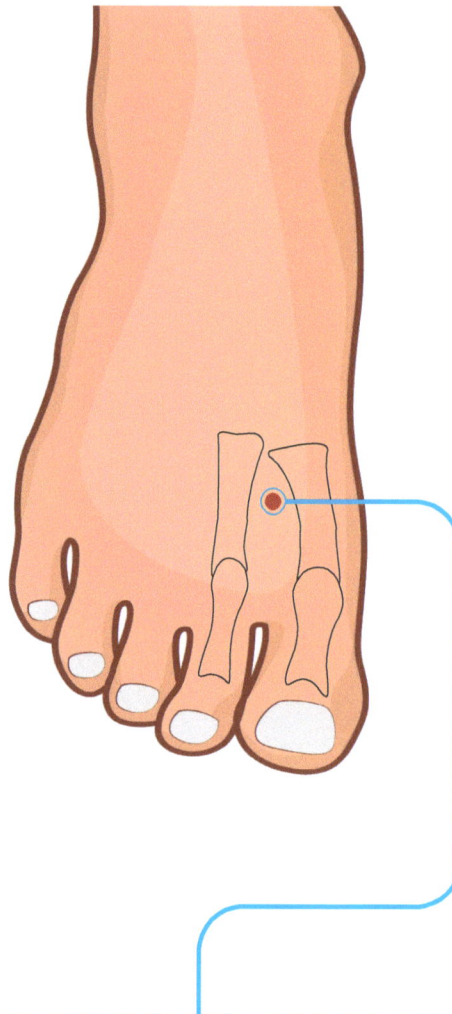

Kabd Thaalith

Location: This area is the region approaching the intersection of the first and second metatarsal bones.

Functions and Indications: It is a very useful area to bleed for all liver disorders and can treat headaches, dizziness, canker sores, blurred vision, red, swollen, painful eyes, dysmennorrhea, amenorrhea, PMS, breast tenderness, anger, irritability, insomnia, anxiety. It is an important point to "descend" qudra in the body.

Method: After making a few small incisions with a blade or lancet, a small cup can be used here though caution is advised if the patient shows signs of liver blood deficiency in which case less blood should be removed.

CORRECT

WRONG

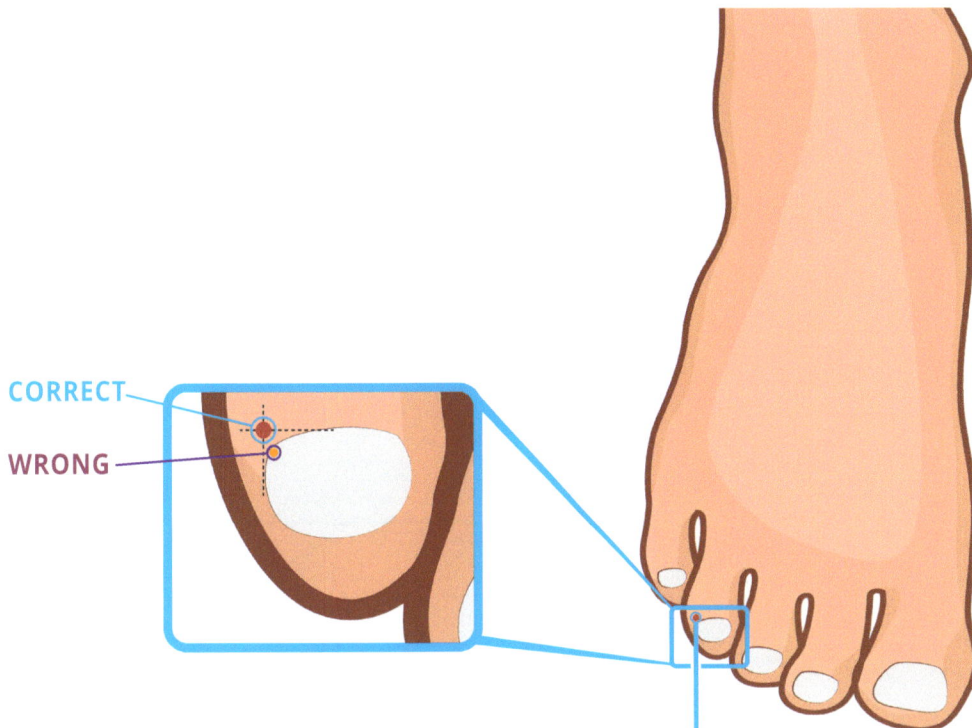

Foot gate - بوابة القدم

Location: At the lateral corner of the 4th toe.

Functions and Indications: Treats Insomnia especially with nightmares caused by heat in the liver and gallbladder rising and affecting the brain. Issues with the sense organs (eyes, ears, nose, mouth, tongue) related to excess heat and/or stagnation - pain, inflammation, speech disorders, stiff tongue.

Method: This point is very sensitive to bleeding and is therefore only used in acute emergency cases. It is bled with a lancet or surgical blade without a cup being applied. Between 2 to 5 drops of blood are squeezed out after making the incision.

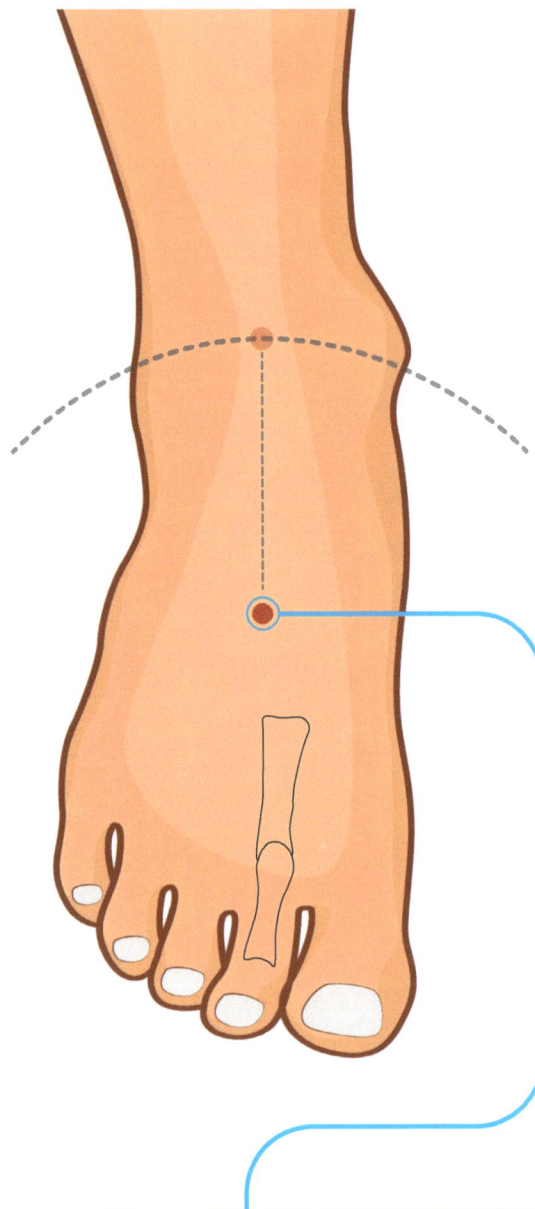

Surging blood - ارتفاع الدم

Location: This point is located on the dorsum of the foot between the 2nd and 3rd metatarsals and the cuneiform bone, between the tendons of the long extensor muscles of the big toe and other toes. While this its typical location, the area descends generally about 2 to 3 finger breadths from this point.

Functions and Indications: Use for the treatment of heat affecting the upper mouth/teeth, toothache, deviation of the face as in bell's palsy or stroke and also for local foot pain, swelling or redness - also for motor control issues of the foot.

Method: Make a few small incisions with a blade or lancet and draw blood with a small cup.

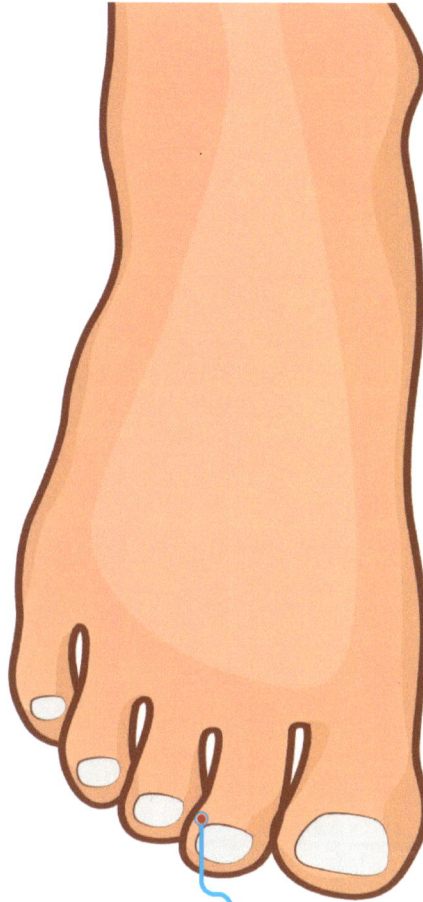

Stomach fire point

Location: 2mm posterior to the corner of the nail on the lateral side of the 2nd toe.

Functions and Indications: Release heat a/or move stagnation from the stomach organ and meridian - Treats headaches, toothaches, facial pain, sore throat, TMJ, bell's palsy, facial deviation from stroke.
Agitation a/or insomnia w/heat signs, excessive dreaming, loss of consciousness, manic depression - calms the mind. All these must be due to heat or fire.

Method: This point is very sensitive to bleeding and is therefore only used in acute emergency cases. It is bled with a lancet or surgical blade without a cup being applied. Between 2 to 5 drops of blood are squeezed out after making the incision.

ظهر القدم

Location: The general area on the anterior aspect of the foot

Functions and indications: This is a point that is recorded in the ahadeeth as being used by the Prophet ﷺ for pain in the same area. This shows is that a point which is painful can be used as well for Hijama

Method: Make incisions with a lancet or blade being careful to avoid the blood vessels in the area and apply a small to medium cup to draw

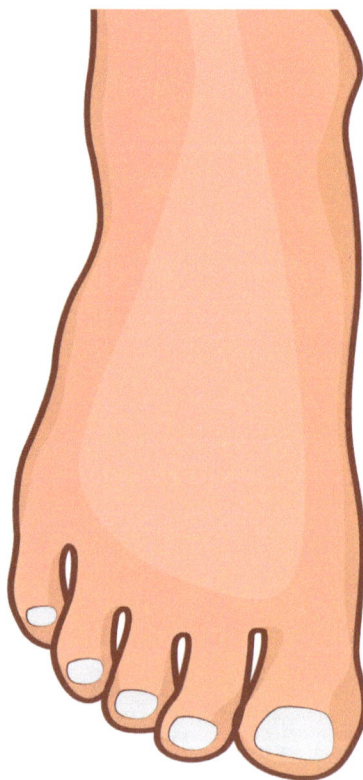

Behind the knee

Location: In the center of the popliteal crease behind the knee

Functions and Indications: This point is connected to the lower back and is used to treat lower back pain due to injury. The pain is characterised by sharp, stabbing pain that may affect the ability of the patient to bed their back. It can also be used for bladder and kidney disorders due to excess such as infections, kidney stones with severe pain and blockage of urine (not due to weakness as in the elderly). Also useful for general heat conditions such as summer heat, heat-stroke and heat exhaustion. Also very effective for all excess skin related issues such as itching, oozing, inflammation and eczema

Method: Check for a small superficial vein in the center or near the center of the crease. If the vein is near the skin and is not thick then it can be pierced directly and this will be very effective for treating pain in the lower back. Alternatively use a lancet to make 3 to 5 incisions and apply a cup to draw blood. The patients knee should be relaxed for the procedure, this can be done by placing a pillow underneath the feet so that the knee is in a relaxed position

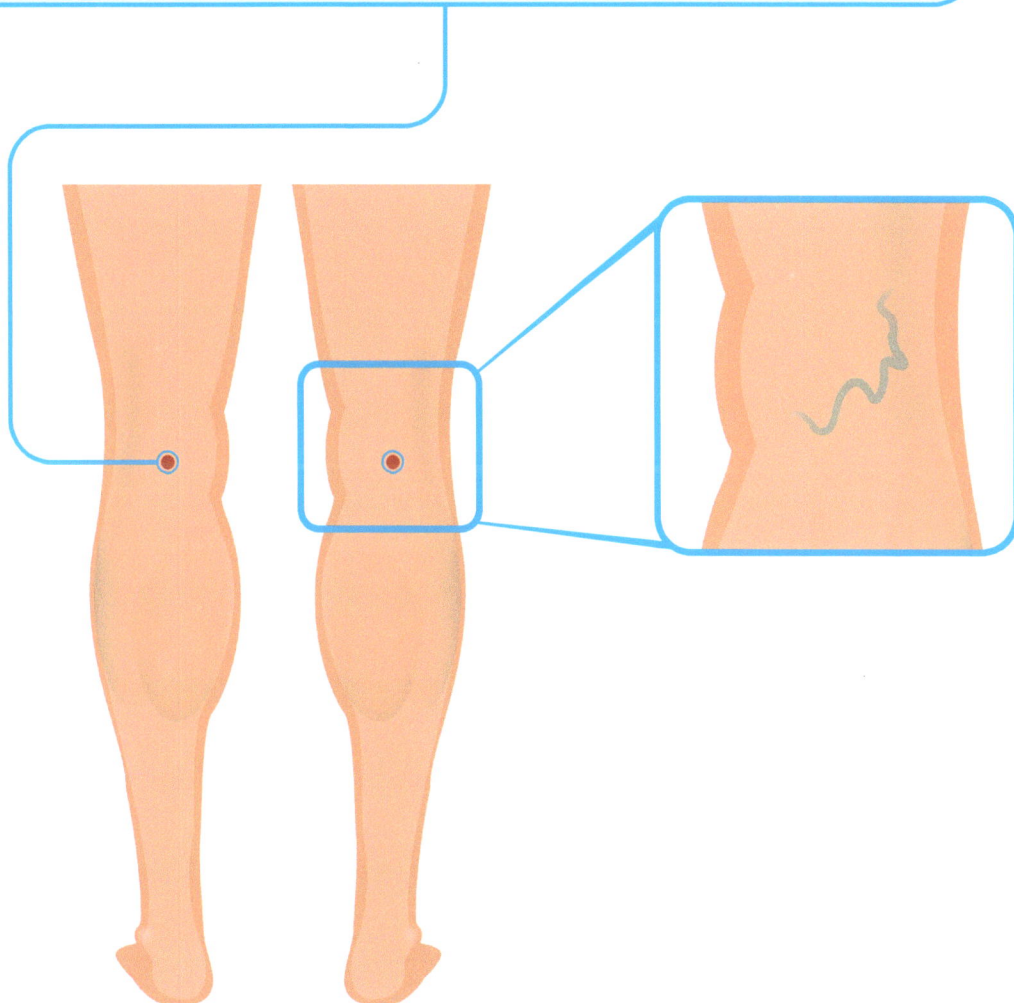

Sea of blood

Location: With the knee flexed, 2.5 finger breadths above the superior medial border of the patella on the bulge of the medial portion of quadriceps femoris (vastus medialis).

Functions and Indications: This point specifically treats gynecological issues originating from Blood stagnation and Heat, maifesting in irregular menstruation, dysmenorrhea, amenorrhea, cramping, UTIs, PMS, uterine bleeding.
Also used for Skin problems due to dampness and heat or hot Blood resulting in eczema, and painful hot skin lesions.
This point is also known to treat genital issues such as pain, swelling or itching of the scrotum or genitals.

Method: Make 5 to 7 incisions with a lancet or surgical blade and apply a medium to large cup to draw blood.

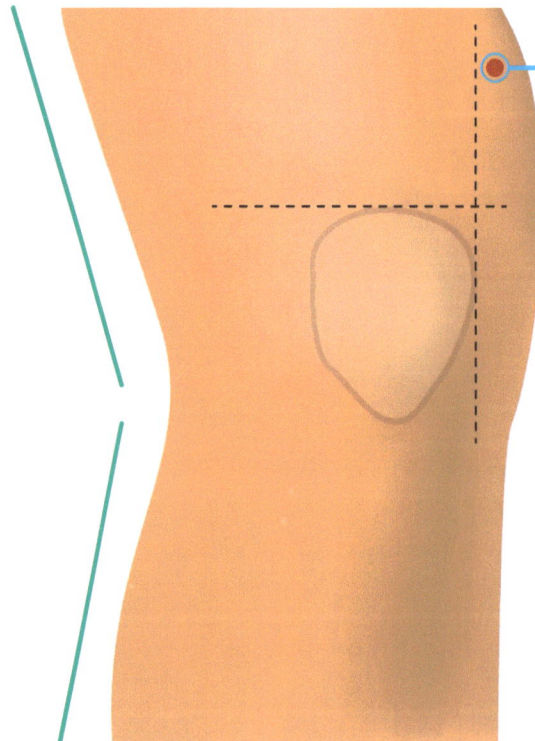

Urinary infection point

Location: 8 finger breadths above the sea of blood point on the lateral side of the sartorius muscle.

Functions and Indications: Used for a variety of urinary issues related to a excess of dampness or dampness with heat in the urinary system.

Indications: Difficult urination, obstruction to urine flow, retention of urine. Also used for swelling in the groin and pain or itching of the external genitalia.

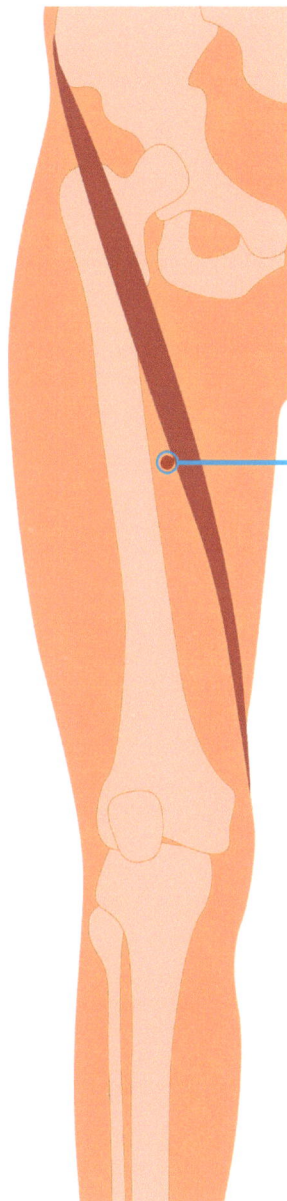

Dry damp point

Location: On the lower border of the medial condyle of the tibia in the depression posterior and inferior to the medial condyle of the tibia. (or) On the lower border of the medial condyle of the tibia on level with the tuberosity of the tibia. (or) Between the posterior border of the tibia and gastrocnemius muscle.

Functions: Dries dampness and swelling especially from the lower body

Indications: Treats any water issue in the body (bloating, swelling, urinary issues, dry mouth, etc.) that is due to an excess factor. Chronic yeast infections, candida. Medial Knee Pain. Issues involving dampness and heat in the gallbladder. Treats hepatitis and jaundice.

Method: Make 3 to 5 incisions with a lancet or surgical blade and apply a small cup to draw blood.

Important: If the swelling or dampness is due to a deficiency factor then do not bleed the point, rather use dry cupping or a different method such as the application of heat or laser (for information on these therapies see courses.drlatib.com)

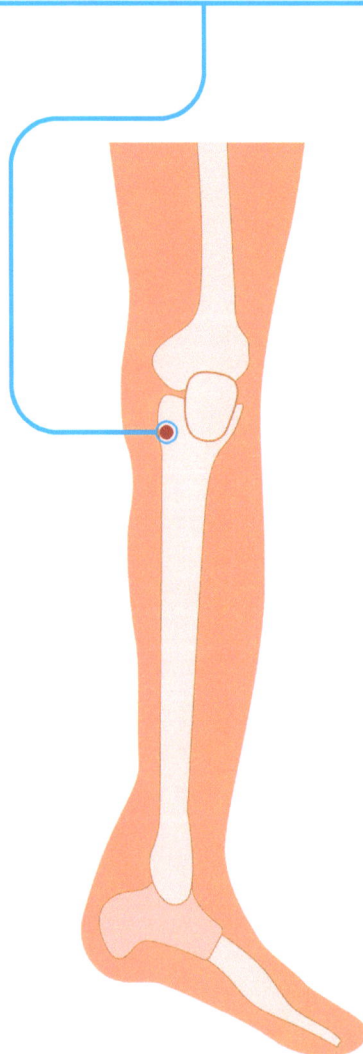

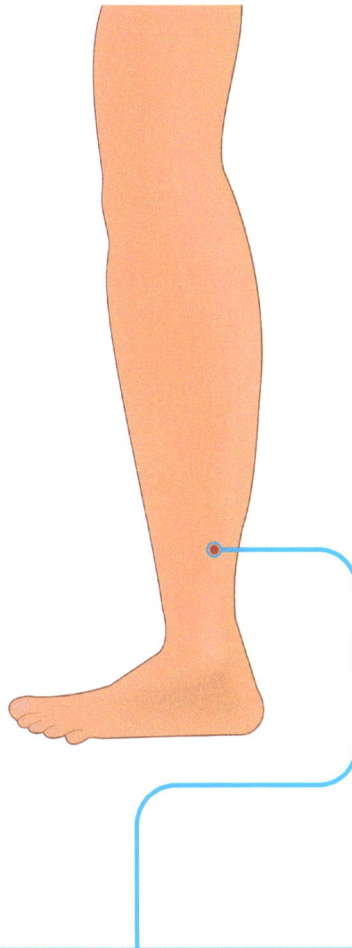

Bone and marrow point

Location: 4 fingers above the tip of the external malleolus in a depression between the posterior border of the fibula and the tendons of peroneous longus and brevis

Functions: Clears excess from the bone marrow and treats the neck, also lowers rising Liver and gallbladder heat.

Indications: Treats excess conditions affecting the bone marrow, ligaments, tendons, muscles or bones resulting in pain, spasms, numbness, weakness. Treats chronic bone and joint pains and wasting if due to excess (if there is a deficiency nature to the illness use dry cupping instead)
Useful for neck issues, stiffness, arthritis, strain, sprain, whiplash, headache.
Also treats dizziness, headache and tinnitus due to liver and gallbladder heat.

Method: Make 3 to 5 small incisions with a surgical blade or lancets and use a small cup to draw blood.

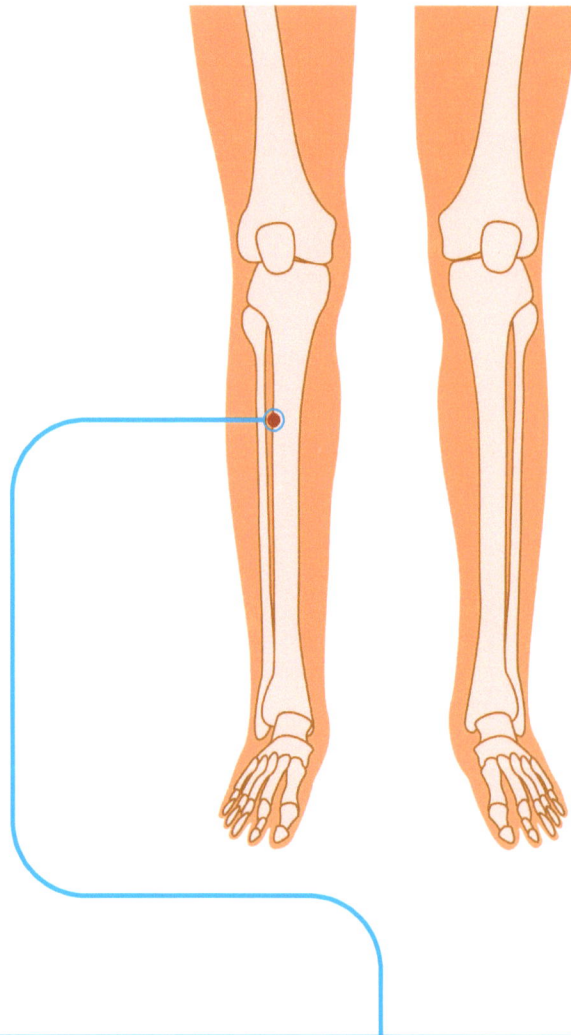

Appendix point

Location: On the right leg only located 6 finger widths down from the bottom of your knee cap, along the outer boundary of your shin bone. This point will be sensitive to pressure if the appendix is inflamed.

Functions and Indications: Used for acute or chronic appendicitis or enteritis

Method: Make 3 to 5 incisions with a lancet and allow to bleed or use a small cylindrical cup to draw blood.

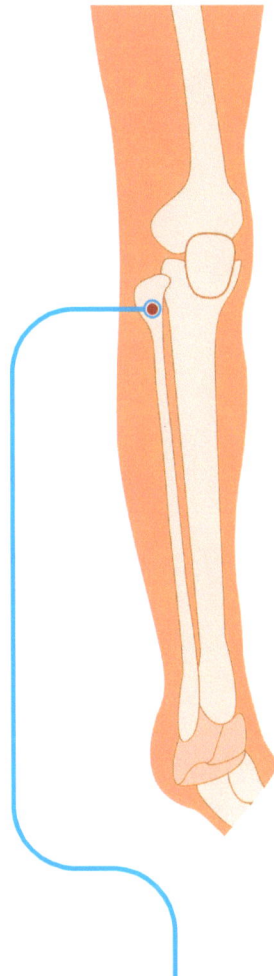

Gallbladder inflammation point

Location: 1.5 to 3 fingerbreadths below the tendon connection point on the right leg only

Functions and Indications: Treats acute cholecystitis, gall stones, post-surgical gallbladder removal pain

Method: Make 3 to 5 incisions with a lancet and allow to bleed or use a small cylindrical cup to draw blood.

Knee eyes

Location: Two points on each knee in the depressions below the patella.

Functions: Treats all knee disorders

Method: Make 3 incisions in each point with a lancet or surgical blade and apply a small to medium cup over

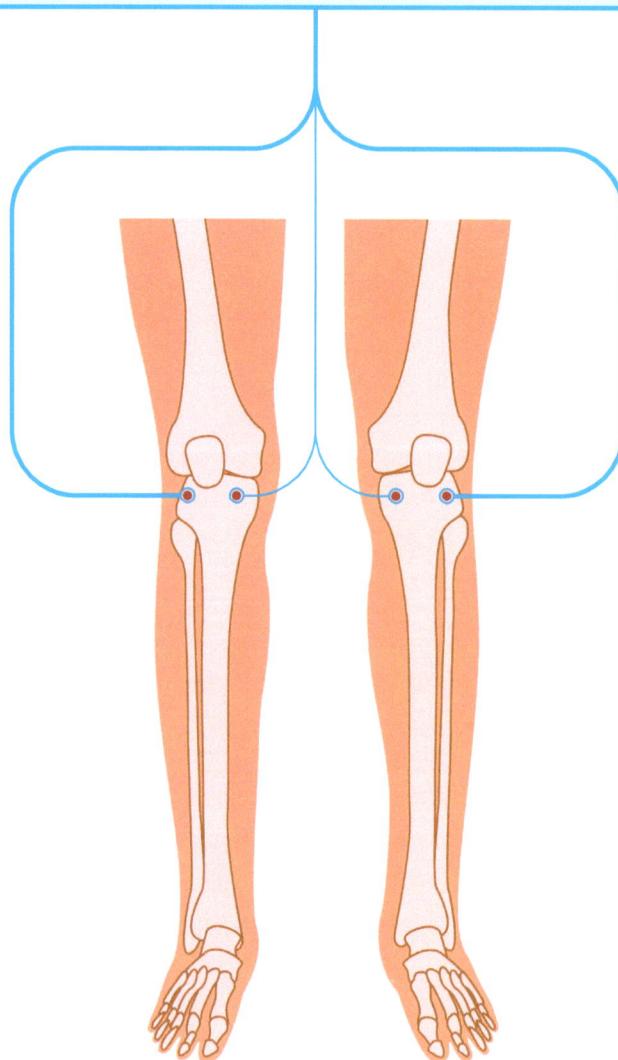

Top of the knee

Location: In a depression at the midpoint of and superior to the patella.

Functions and indications: Treats all knee disorders

Method: Make 3 incisions in each point with a lancet or surgical blade and apply a small to medium cup over

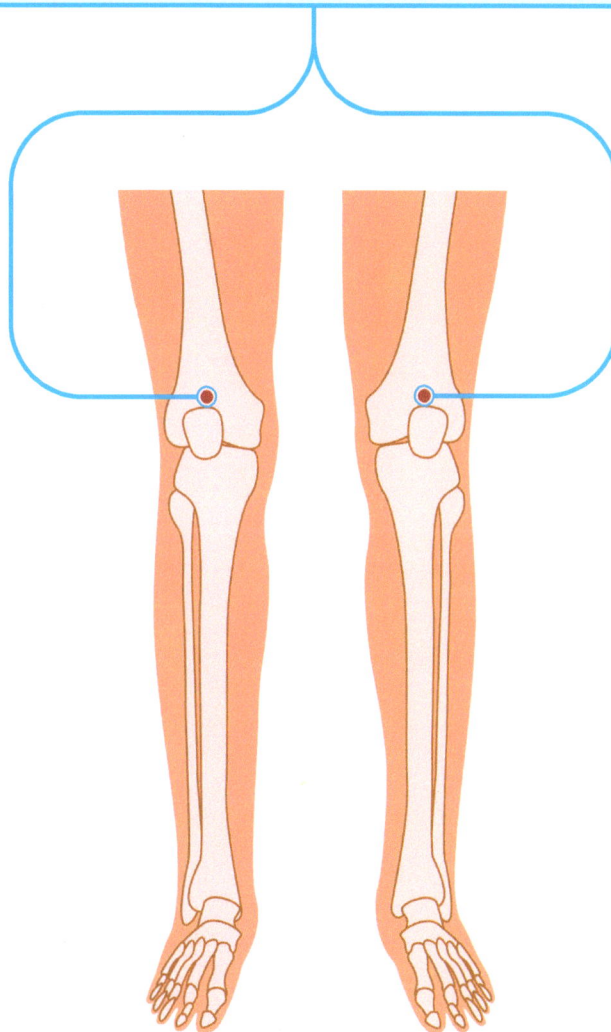

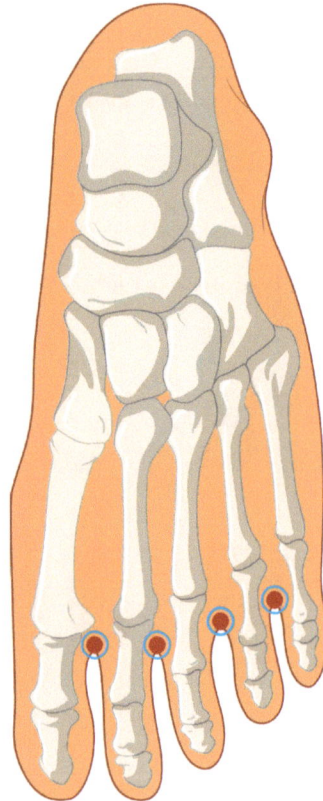

Foot malaria points

Location: On the dorsum of the foot between the web and metatarsophalangeal joint (4 points on each foot).

Functions and Indications: Treats malaria and malaria type fevers

Method: Bleed each point with a lancet or surgical blade and allow to bleed

You will find that while studying this manual that there are often multiple Hijama points that can be used for the same illness. The question will then arise as to which point or points will be best to use, or would you use all of them in the same session. Point selection strategy in itself is an area of study and without guidance it is difficult to know what is the preferred method.

There are a number of considerations that need to be made when selecting points, I have detailed them below under the two main divisions of Hijama therapy:

General (health maintenance) Hijama

When performing general Hijama which is intended for health maintenance or the control of excess heat that can arise due to living in a hot climate:

1. The points selected will be primarily those that are recorded in the hadeeth as used for this purpose, viz. the upper back region and the occipital and scalp region.

2. The constitution of the patient must be assessed, if the constitution is strong then 4 to 6 different points can be bled

3. The head should generally only be used if the patient complains of headaches.

4. The occipital and upper shoulder regions can be used if the patient complains of muscle stiffness in this area

5. If it is the first time that the patient is having Hijama and they are of weak constitution or apprehensive of the procedure then use 2 to 4 points only

Hijama for specific illnesses

There are more considerations and guidelines when using Hijama for a specific illness and they are as follows:-

1. If it is an emergency condition such as loss of consciousness, extremely high fever, convulsions or epilepsy, heatstroke etc then the "tips" are most effective, viz the fingertip points, the points at the corners of the nails, the ear apex point etc.

2. If it is a chronic condition the points on the back are generally the most effective.

3. If you are treating a patient over a period of multiple sessions then the points on the back and the front can be alternated at each session so that the effectiveness of the therapy is improved while the same points are not being bled continuously

4. It is good to combine points on the extremities (which normally require removing a few drops) together with points on the torso, this enhances effectiveness

5. Sometimes you have to take into account that if you are a male treating a female patient, in the presence of another person always, then it will be preferred to use points that do not require revealing more of the skin than is necessary

6. Being able to identify and correctly diagnose heat, cold, excess, deficiency, stagnation, stasis and the state of the organs and body fluids will allow you to select and use the points much more effectively. This can be learnt through the courses at my website www.drlatib.com

With experience you will begin to identify which points are more effective for which condition and stage of illness إن شاء الله تعالى

May Allah ﷻ make you a means of shifaa (cure) for thousands of people, Aameen

Dr Feroz Osman-Latib

www.ingramcontent.com/pod-product-compliance
Lightning Source LLC
Chambersburg PA
CBHW040713280326
41926CB00083B/47